Confronting Malice

Confronting Malice

*A Memoir of Working
with Sex and Violent Offenders*

ANNA C. SALTER

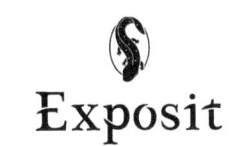

Exposit

Jefferson, North Carolina

"Lyin' Eyes," words and Music by Don Henley and Glenn Frey. Copyright © 1975 CASS COUNTY MUSIC and RED LOUD MUSIC. Copyright Renewed. All Rights Administered by UNIVERSAL MUSIC WORKS. All Rights Reserved. Used by Permission. *Reprinted by Permission of Hal Leonard LLC.*

"Live," from *Live or Die*, by Anne Sexton. Reprinted by permission of SLL/Sterling Lord Literistic, Inc. Copyright by Linda Gray Sexton.

"Man Carrying Thing," copyright © 1954 by Wallace Stevens and copyright renewed 1982 by Holly Stevens; from THE COLLECTED POEMS OF WALLACE STEVENS by Wallace Stevens. Used by permission of Alfred A. Knopf, an imprint of the Knopf Doubleday Publishing Group, a division of Penguin Random House LLC. All rights reserved.

"The Summer Day," by Mary Oliver. Reprinted by permission of The Charlotte Sheedy Literary Agency as agent for the author. Copyright © 1900, 2006, 2008, 2017 by Mary Oliver with permission of Bill Reichblum.

"Tired of London" (poem), *Light Me Down: The New & Collected Poems of Jean Valentine* by Jean Valentine, Alice James Books, 2024.

ISBN (print) 978-1-4766-9689-8
ISBN (ebook) 978-1-4766-5621-2

LIBRARY OF CONGRESS CATALOGING DATA ARE AVAILABLE

© 2025 Anna C. Salter. All rights reserved

No part of this book may be reproduced or transmitted in any form or by any means, electronic or mechanical, including photocopying or recording, or by any information storage and retrieval system, without permission in writing from the publisher.

Front cover photograph by Marco Tiberio (Shutterstock)

Printed in the United States of America

Exposit is an imprint of McFarland & Company, Inc., Publishers

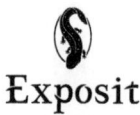

Exposit

Box 611, Jefferson, North Carolina 28640
www.expositbooks.com

For Ellie and Alegrar.
Each of whom brings joy
in their own way

Acknowledgments

I would like to thank Sandi Gelles Coles, who has been my editor since my first mysteries. It is rare to run into someone who is creative, thoughtful, loyal, and ethical, all qualities she exudes.

Thanks to my friend Jennifer Hoult, who reads all my works, and they are far better for her thoughts. A Renaissance woman, she is brilliant in every field she takes up.

I want to thank Alegrar, who lives up to his name.

My friend Geri Crisci has kept me at least semi sane for more than 20 years. She is the lighthouse that keeps me off most rocks.

Table of Contents

Acknowledgments   vi
Preface   1
Introduction   3

Chapter 1. The Coliseum   11
Chapter 2. Beginnings   16
Chapter 3. On Malice   25
Chapter 4. Nemesis   31
Chapter 5. The Country Doc   43
Chapter 6. How Psychopaths Think   52
Chapter 7. Working with Psychopaths   63
Chapter 8. The Interview   73
Chapter 9. On Feeling Safe: Where Does Safety Lie?   84
Chapter 10. Grief for a Lost Son   93
Chapter 11. Three Years Later   102
Chapter 12. On Connection   108
Chapter 13. On Being Safe: Guns and Poses   114
Chapter 14. The Social Contract   121
Chapter 15. Homes and Houses   135
Chapter 16. Hope   144
Chapter 17. On the Problem with Power   150
Chapter 18. The Conman and the Courts   158

Table of Contents

Chapter 19. Society and Sex Offenders — 172
Chapter 20. Lessons — 179

Epilogue — 183
Chapter Notes — 187
Bibliography — 189

Preface

This book has been growing since I first began to work with sex and violent offenders, 40 years ago. The worldview of the offenders I interviewed seemed so alien to me that I felt I had gone through the rabbit hole and was now a co-inhabitant of Alice's land. I did not understand the callousness, the malevolence, and the indifference of the highest risk offenders that I worked with. For better or worse, I have maintained much of that sense of incredulity, but I do know things now I would never have known without those 40 years. I know what it takes to survive in court, what it is like to interview people who make a habit of harming others (sometimes fatally), where malice comes from, the motivations and thought processes of child molesters, what is missing in psychopaths, the difference in a home and a house. This book explores what took me down that rabbit hole, what I learned while there, and what it is like to climb out and leave the world of deviancy and malevolence behind.

I am a frayed and nibbled survivor in a fallen world,
and I am getting along.
—Annie Dillard, *Pilgrim at Tinker Creek*

Introduction

> "What is it you plan to do
> with your one wild and precious life?"
> —Mary Oliver, "The Summer Day"[1]

    I didn't start out wanting to be a sex offender evaluator and therapist, a trainer and speaker on all things dark and dreadful. I wanted to be Bill Russell when I grew up. I wanted to play for the Celtics. I spent every day in the summer in a tiny Southern gym which, no doubt, reached 100 degrees regularly. After team practice in the winter, I went home and played by myself for three more hours.
    Oddly, the Celtics never called, missing their chance to add a 5'6" guard to their roster, and somehow it has come to this: I have spent 40 years studying, assessing, and treating sex and violent offenders and their victims. I have been in court well over 200 times. I have done trainings in 10 countries and multiple times in all 50 states. I have traveled well over a million miles by air, over 800,000 on one airline alone. I am actually over one-third of the way to my second million although I don't expect (or want) to make it. Like Dave Barry, I want the kind of frequent flier program where, with enough miles, you get to stay home. I know I have spent more time in motels than most prostitutes, as they have shorter careers. I have made films on sex offenders that were posted on YouTube and, depending on the film or the film clip, have gathered anywhere from 500,000 to 3.5 million views. In the last 10 years alone, I have assessed at least 425 sexually violent offenders. At one point, I had a two-year period during which I testified in four trials where children and youth had killed their parents (three) or a complete stranger (one). One year I

Introduction

testified in three different torture trials in three weeks. I have written three nonfiction books on sex offenders and five mysteries. The mysteries kept me going; in fiction, the good guys always win. Too, the mysteries gave an outlet to Michael, the female protagonist. Much was made in reviews of her name as some sort of cross-sex reference, but the reality was, she was simply named for a female friend of mine I admired who worked in the same field, and my friend's name was literally Michael.

The Michael of my mysteries said all the things I wanted to say but was too professional to voice. She was a smart-ass, and while sharp retorts and rebukes went through my head continually—after all, what would you think when someone said, "I slipped on the stairs and fell down them. She was at the bottom and my pants came undone and my penis landed in her mouth" as a way to explain a child's report of oral sex—for the most part I managed to color within the lines and restrict my sense of outrage to my head and the pages of my novels.

The mysteries didn't sell enough to keep publishers interested, but even if they had, somewhere along the way I lost Michael, and I don't think I could have kept writing them. I kept changing, and the smart-ass comments in my head became less funny and more exasperated and indignant. Somehow preaching in outrage is not the same thing as writing a good mystery. Michael, for all her flaws, was more hopeful than I became. But my whole path into the world of deviancy and crime was an accident anyway.

Had you asked that 14-year-old girl playing basketball in her backyard and dreaming of being Bill Russell if she was going to work with sex offenders when she grew up, you would likely have heard "huh?" The "huh?" would have continued had you asked in college or in either of the two graduate school programs I attended. I never had a course on child abuse in my 23 years of schooling up through a doctorate. I never even had a lecture. But, once I graduated with my Ph.D. and went to work in a small community mental health center, it seemed that every other child who came in had been sexually,

Introduction

physically, or emotionally abused or neglected. I did what I could to adapt the techniques I was taught for working with children who had other issues but threw up my hands when the court started sending sex offenders to the clinic for treatment that I worked at instead of to jail. I had no idea how to assess or treat these people.

I have been asked why I didn't turn my back on this type of client and refuse to see them. But I was working in a community mental health center and not a private practice. You saw who came through the door. It was a small community, and we were the only mental health center so when you were up for the next intake, you took whoever walked or was dragged in. And too, here was an opportunity to do something that might actually be useful: prevent small children and adults from being raped and molested. Maybe I should have said no, but I didn't. Instead, I wrote and received a small grant from the State of Vermont to go around the country looking at programs that treated sex offenders and to then write up some guidelines for the State of Vermont. I found a treatment program called Northwest Treatment Associates in Seattle, Washington, that seemed comprehensive and more effective than others I visited. With their permission, I wrote up the techniques they used and even included the homework assignments. But the report I was writing just kept growing and growing, and it ended up becoming my first book: *Treating Child Sex Offenders and Victims: A Practical Guide*, published in 1988. There was so little information available on sex offenders and victims in 1988 that the book seemed to go everywhere. I ended up lecturing as far away as Australia and New Zealand on that book. And so, a path opened up that I never expected. I began to assess and treat sex offenders. At first, I saw many more victims than offenders, but over time, the fact that many more people wanted to work with victims than offenders meant the need was greater in the offender world, and I was steadily drawn into it.

One of the questions I get asked most when I do trainings is how I got into this field. When I describe the serendipity that altered the course of my life, no one is ever satisfied. It is as though people believe

Introduction

that lives and career paths follow straight lines, that we choose the worlds we work in entirely according to our inner needs. No doubt our proclivities and interests play a role, but sometimes they dictate the process more than the content of our choices. My father was a country doc. He lived a life of purpose, and he imbued me with the sense that a life of purpose was the most satisfying way to live. But being a medical doctor was out for me. When I was age five, he suggested I might want to be a doctor when I grew up, and I replied that I didn't like sores on my body or anyone else's. I still remember being asked to cut up a living earthworm in a biology class in high school. It's a traumatic memory.

But preventing child abuse by assessing and treating offenders: that I could do. So, when the opportunity came along, I didn't run screaming into the desert. I believed, and still believe, that it is better to prevent children from becoming victims than to try to undo the damage afterward.

Working with offenders involved court, of course, and many psychologists will absolutely not go into any subspecialty where going to court is even a possibility. But I grew up fighting with an emotionally abusive mother, and too, from seventh grade on, I was elbowing boys under the boards in a rural Southern gym. I expected to have to fight.

I stayed too because the thinking patterns of offenders fascinated me. I could obsess more on forgetting to send a thank you note than some of the offenders I have talked to worried about committing triple murder. In fact, one man who killed his grandmother and two boarders who happened to be home at the time told me that if he hadn't have done that, he wouldn't be the man he was today. He evidently felt that triple murder was a character-building experience. Garrison Keillor captured this kind of thinking perfectly in an essay called "The Current Crisis in Remorse" in his book *We Are Still Married.*

> People in the helping professions had noticed a dramatic increase in the number of clients who did terrible things and didn't feel one bit sorry.

Introduction

> It was an utterly common phenomenon for a man who had been apprehended after months of senseless carnage to look at a social worker or psychologist with an expression of mild dismay and say, "Hey, I know what you are thinking, but that wasn't *me* out there, it wasn't *like* me at all. I'm a caring kind of guy. Anyway, it's over now, it's done, and I got to get on with my own life, you know," as if he had only been unkind or unsupportive of his victims and not dismembered them and stuffed them into mailboxes [Keillor, 1982].

Keillor thought he was joking, but I have spoken with offenders who, almost word for word, made the same statements. The thinking, the rationales, the excuses, the values (or lack of them) were all just so *strange*, so *odd*. I wanted to understand the forces that drove these men, their motivations, their thinking patterns. A professor of mine at Harvard once said in a lecture, "When smart people do stupid things, powerful forces are at work." The same could be said for immoral things. I wanted to understand the powerful forces. So, I stayed.

But in the process, my old worldview began to seem like a mirage. I changed, often in sad ways that could not be redeemed. I don't think like most people anymore. I've seen too many "people of the lie." They aren't all in prison. More often, they move freely among us, paying nothing for the privilege of predation. Too many times, I have asked a victim what happened to the author of a particularly brutal rape, and she has looked at me in astonishment and said, "Nothing," as though no other outcome was conceivable. "He's[2] still ..." and the rest of the sentence could be anything: running the fire department, moderating the town meeting, teaching at the high school—or the elementary school—living a comfortable life after retiring from the parish. The rest of the sentence will describe an unruffled life that proceeded as if the victims he made were deadwood tossed up on the beach, insignificant and quickly forgotten.

Certainly, there are offenders falsely convicted and that is a tragedy. I once told a prosecutor in an appeals case that he was wrong, that the adolescent in question had made a false confession under pressure—and got thanked and thrown off the case for

Introduction

my trouble. My opinion isn't for sale, just my time in forming it. I have always turned down cases I didn't believe in. But the other side is there also: how many offenders in prison or in civil commitment talk—sometimes brag—about cases they were never charged with or where they were falsely acquitted? Of the offenders I have assessed who have been in treatment, most ended up admitting many more undetected or acquitted offenses than they were caught for.

I am not saying that all who commit sexual or violent crimes have made malevolence a way of life. There are lost souls out there whose crimes are errors in judgment or impulsive acts by the young and the rash. But make no mistake, malice exists. Not every violent person who says he or she is sorry means it. Not every person who says he won't do it again is even planning on making an effort. What I am saying is that the average layperson—and, frankly, most professionals—can't tell the difference between a sinner and a psychopath, between those who made a mistake and those for whom offending is "better than crack, better than cocaine." Am I infallible in my ability to discern? Hardly. But 40 years buys you something.

But I am not writing this to tell war stories and blow off steam. That is too easy and too intellectually cheap. I am writing to make sense of the men who commit sexual violence, to understand the differences between the lost and the malevolent, and also to make sense of my own journey and how the forces in my childhood made working in this field for 40 years even possible. Too, I am writing to make sense of people's reactions to offenders. Sex offenders are an abstract group of demons to most people—unless they happen to know one of them. If it's Cousin Stevie, then it's a shame he made a mistake, and he won't do it again—if he did it in the first place, which he probably didn't.

I understand. Attachment makes deniers of us all. It softens the critical faculties until the word "evidence" no longer has any meaning: there is never enough proof if you love someone. But even if

Introduction

Stevie isn't a cousin, even if he's the art teacher in the local school and they've never met him, it's nonetheless easy to convince a jury that an adolescent victim is a lying little twerp. We need to feel safe, and the possibility that *an art teacher in a local public school is a sex offender* doesn't make for sleep that will stitch up any raveled sleeves.

I thought about writing a book on violence without reference to my own history, without giving a thought to what has allowed me to do the work I do and how it has reverberated in my life. But total objectivity is not quite a false god, but surely an imperfect one. We all see life through the lens of our own minds, informed by our past and our present. "The past is never dead," Faulkner famously wrote. "In fact, it is not even past." I would only add it is sometimes more alive than the present. It is the lens through which we see the present, informing what we *can* see and how we see it.

When I tried to keep the book strictly professional, it wilted in my hands. It only came alive for me when I interwove my story with the work I do. And that's the problem with books. Authors really don't have complete control of them. Writing is a game of warmer, colder. Get too mechanistic and you'll end up with frozen hands. You can write a sentence, and it may be fine stylistically; it may even be clever. But if the writer is left cold by it, it's worthless. Books have more control over where they want to go than you think.

"Trust your unconscious," Milton Erickson wrote. "It knows more than you do" (Erickson, 2017). The writer who lives in my head sees things I don't and makes sense of things I puzzle over. There is the unformed sea in all our heads edging up to the formed sand, the words on the page. That line—the one between the sea and the shore—the line between the unformed and the formed—is where I write. It's where all authors write. I write in perpetual surprise to see the thoughts that I often didn't know I had. Who lives back there in my head? Beats me, but I try to stay on good terms with her. I write to find out what *she* thinks. Wallace Stevens wrote, "We must endure our thoughts all night, until / The bright obvious stands motionless in cold" (Stevens, 1990).

Introduction

Any author will tell you that when books want to be written they will drive you crazy. I have three books now poking at me in various ways. One is a book on how the memory and suggestibility research gets misused in court in child sexual abuse cases. That book is tugging at my sleeve. Another book, on what I have learned in over 400 interviews in the last few years, is humming in the background. Thus far they have been too polite to get anywhere with me. But this book drove me out of the shower to write a single sentence. It bubbled up in meditation. It made me turn off a *Green Bay Packers game*—which is probably illegal in Wisconsin—to explore a new line of thought. If it hasn't gotten me into a car wreck yet, it has been by the sheerest of margins. You don't write the polite book that wants to be written. You write the rude and demanding book that grabs you by the throat and won't let go until you do.

So, what is this book about? It is about psychopaths and sinners and a gym rat from a small town in North Carolina who somehow ended up with a Ph.D. from Harvard and has spent her entire professional life in small rooms talking to people who rape and molest and sometimes murder people.

But I would argue it is also about one of the most compelling issues of our time: interpersonal violence. It's the thing we have to fix if there is ever going to be peace on this planet. Sure, I know interpersonal violence on an individual level is not the whole story. There are wars and terrorists, climate disaster, and murder on the scale of genocide. But person-to-person violence in the form of crime changes millions of lives for the worse each year. There are few of us who don't know someone who has been molested or raped or mugged or hurt violently in some way by a fellow human being. They say if it ain't broke, don't fix it. Well, this is broke. And the route to fixing it lies, first of all, in making sense of it. For better or worse, I have tried to do that, and here's what the sea tossed up.

Chapter 1

The Coliseum

I am going to court, or, rather, the Coliseum. After all, this is where paid professionals duke it out. I have on my Dr. Anna clothes: the obligatory suit jacket, this time over a black dress. I wear the same low heels I have for 10 years. Well, they're comfortable. I am wearing jewelry. I am wearing make-up. The aging jock who spends every possible moment in jeans and a turtleneck is gone. Dr. Anna is back.

They say that court is the only contact sport left in the social sciences, but it is less a contact sport than a field of land mines. Not only do I have to remember every little detail of the case—which ran to 8,000 pages of records—I have to remember all the judge's rulings: the evidence that has been excluded, the things that the judge has ruled I cannot say. If anything excluded slips out of my mouth, it could mean a mistrial or an issue for appeal that gets the case overturned. That happened once in my four decades of practice, and it nearly killed me.

Then there is the research on which I will base my testimony. I have spent 15 hours just reviewing this literature. This is a child sexual abuse case where the victim did not report right away. Juries tend to distrust delayed disclosure and incorrectly assume it is a sign of a false report. I am bringing a notebook filled with 42 studies on delayed disclosure, and it is indisputable that delayed disclosure is actually the norm; the first impact of sexual abuse is most often silence. Those children who disclose at all often wait years to do so. I have summarized each study so I can refer to it quickly. I have read, organized, and annotated research on the impact of a lack of maternal support, on memory, on suggestibility, on children's conception of time, and on the impact of threats. You do not have to have a diagnosis of obsessive-compulsive disorder to testify as an expert witness, but it helps.

Nonetheless, poring over the research will not get me through the day. It is emotional presence that makes testimony and trainings compelling. It is bringing yourself, all of you as you are at that exact moment, to the stand. It is being *emotionally fresh* that causes jurors to lift their heads and listen. The problem is that on any given day, I can feel any number of ways about testifying, and I do not have enough foresight to figure out in advance how I am going to feel.

Mindfulness, or living in the emotional present, is well known to impact health and well-being. Neurologists swear by it. Google runs classes for its employees. Sports teams practice it. School children are trained with clever games to stay in the moment—which bespeaks an eye-rolling amount of adult arrogance, as it is similar to trying to teach monkeys to climb. But what the books and lectures, internet blogs and posts don't tell you is the impact of emotional mindfulness on people around you. People listen to you when you are not rehearsed, when you are emotionally present, and they don't when you aren't. Everyone feels the difference, from the person two feet away to the person at the back of a 500-person auditorium.

But the problem with mindfulness is that by its very nature you can't anticipate it. You do not decide in advance how you are going to feel at any given moment; you discover it. On this day, I don't figure out where I am and what my relationship with the jury is until I am in the witness box. I am pleased to realize I am not on my soapbox today. I can get on an indignation kick, and that can quickly turn into the fatal error of lecturing the jury. If I am outraged, it will not transfer to the jury. Only if I am calm and objective will the jury be outraged by the case. I am also pleased I do not have to listen to inanity or sheer cruelty by the defense—the lawyer for the defense treated the child courteously, and his questions made sense. I realize where I am today when I look at the jeans and the sneakers of the jury and see

Chapter 1. The Coliseum

the contrast with the suits and high heels of the lawyers, the contrast with the high ceilings, the stiff, ornate furnishings, and the elevated figure in the black robe. Why do courtrooms have such high, grand ceilings? Is justice to be found in grandeur? Does there need to be room up there for someone to look down? We're not allowed to eat or drink. Is no one supposed to gain sustenance here? This is the Himalayan kill zone, where everyone deteriorates over time.

I realize what I feel today is that we together, the jury and I, are going to humanize this inhospitable place. That is my job: to say what I need to say informally as though we are just having a conversation. To look at each juror in turn, to be blessedly brief after all they have had to listen to, to stay away from psychological jargon—which I despise anyway—to make sense of things.

Nonetheless, I have brought my book of studies, my annotated lists, and my bibliographies. I place them carefully on the stand in front of me. It is not for the prosecution or even the jury. The jury could care less about correlation coefficients. It is a statement to the defense: if you want to take me on about whether delayed disclosure is normative, be my guest, but I have worked my butt off to be ready and you will have to know more about these studies than I do.

There is a lot at stake. There is always a lot at stake. This time I am testifying in a torture case. I am testifying for a child who was beaten, removed from school, forced to live in an unheated basement in freezing Wisconsin without a bathroom, forced to eat her feces when she had to defecate, and starved for five years. Her stepmother put her in the basement shortly after the child told a teacher that her half-brother was sexually abusing her. If you're not in school and you're not allowed to go out or have friends, there's no one to tell. She weighed 80 pounds at age 10 when she went in. When she got out at age 15, she weighed 68. Her growth, her cognition, and her social skills are permanently stunted.

The parents are now in prison for torturing her, but they are only there for brief stints. Apparently, torturing a child is worth five years with this judge. Had they done something *serious*—say, steal a car—they might have served longer. Today the antisocial, possibly psychopathic, adolescent stepbrother is on trial for beating and raping the starving child multiple times. This jury will never know it because the evidence has been excluded as prejudicial,[1] but this offender has made a habit of molesting kids. There are three other victims of his in various stages of the legal process.

The prosecutor rises and the dance begins. I lean forward and raise an open face. This isn't difficult. After all, the DA is trying to make me look good. The hard part will come later when I am crossed. Today is a good day on direct. This prosecutor is excellent, and he too has done his homework. He gets everything out of me that I have to offer. Direct today is like riding in a Ferrari. There have been days with other attorneys when I sat bottled up with information but without the questions that would allow me to talk about it. You can't "narrate" as an expert witness; you have to wait for the questions and sometimes the right questions don't come. Sometimes the attorneys forget. Sometimes they don't think it's important. Sometimes we don't agree on what the right questions are. Sometimes I am riding in a car that won't start. They say in sports that you never play a good game against a bad team. Maybe. But in court you can play a good game against a bad team; you just can't play a good game *with* a bad team. Whenever I can get a ride in a Ferrari, I am Grateful Gladys.

The defense attorney rises, and I lean forward with the same open face, the same body language. Even honest expert witnesses make the rookie mistake of looking afraid when cross begins. I have watched other expert witnesses, even fair and impartial experts, recoil in horror when the opposing attorney approaches them. Their brows furrow. They lean back, take a couple of nervous sips of water and look as though a giant snake is slithering across the floor toward them: Nagini's on the loose or perhaps it's Voldemort himself. Of course, they may be right—Nagini may be heading their way—but reacting that way sends a message that the opposing attorney is their enemy, and they are on one side and not an independent and objective witness.

Chapter 1. The Coliseum

An effective expert witness must telegraph to the jury that she is simply an expert in her field providing objective and balanced information to the court. She is happy to answer anybody's questions. Of course, the opposing attorney is not likely to treat her that way: the lawyer walking toward her is going to try to make her look like an idiot, no matter how fair and balanced she is, and it's natural to have some dread when you know someone is going to try to twist your words. But that's the job of the defense. The lawyers for the defendant don't have to be fair and balanced. They are just trying to win, and it's only human to feel trepidation at the sound of the slithering. And even if Nagini is heading your way, a lean forward, a small smile and a cloudless face are as important as the suit and the heels. They also have the added advantage of getting you in the right mindset. Despite the fact that the opposing attorney is trying to make you look like a hired gun, you don't actually have to be one. In truth you *are* there to present fair and balanced information to the court, and the body language helps keep you in that mindset. I might add that as a bonus it infuriates the opposing attorney who is hoping to get you into a pissing match.[2]

Humor is iffy in court and can rarely be used without risk but once, and only once, when an attorney was screaming at me, I tried it. I had been responding to his tactics with my standard, puzzled look: "Why on earth," the look said, "is he acting this way?" which is exactly how I felt, but he made one hostile and demeaning statement too many. As he turned his back to walk back to the table, I turned to the jury and shrugged. The jury burst into laughter, and the attorney whipped around to see what happened. There wasn't any way for him to find out. I never tried humor again. Go out on top.

Later I wait for the text from the prosecution. It takes the jury 10 hours, but they do figure out he's guilty. It is 12:20 a.m. before I get the news and relief floods over me. No one has to tell this child, who has already lived through hell, that the jury didn't believe her.

Chapter 2

Beginnings

Self Portrait

At best, it is the face of a racehorse
Pale with intelligence
Carved clean with the fear of losing
Bold
With that deep stubbornness
Found in thoroughbreds
And Southerners
And brain-damaged children

The problem with that poem, which I wrote over 40 years ago, is that I'm not sure where I fit on that continuum. Southerner, for sure. But it gets dicey after that.

Where did this stubbornness come from? If nothing else, I am tenacious and downright stubborn on the stand. I do my best to hide it: the cloudless face, the polite answers—I am trying to come across as a reasonable person. But a mistake that many expert witnesses make is to agree with the opposing attorney when they don't really agree—just to avoid conflict, to avoid being attacked. They will swallow their opinions and take back their assessments. Most of us aren't geared for battle. We are programmed to keep the social blanket that spreads between us smooth and unruffled. But I am not built like that. It's not that I'm looking for conflict on the stand. It's just inevitable. No matter how good your assessment, no matter how many studies your opinion is based on, the opposing attorney's job is to attack it and you. You could say Earth is round and s/he'd be at your throat. "It's not *exactly* round, now, is it, doctor?"

This degree of stubbornness is not always an asset. It is a near

Chapter 2. Beginnings

disaster in social relationships and a total disaster in marriage. (Married twice; divorced twice.) I have had to learn the long, hard way to keep a close rein on my stubbornness outside the legal arena. Mostly I can do it. Clay Matthews didn't run around tackling people once he stepped off the football field. You just have to channel it.

Looking back, I can't remember ever not being stubborn. Or being without that strange trait where I just don't accept other people's opinions all that easily. It leaked out everywhere. As a young child, I didn't realize that I had done anything wrong when I asked the Sunday School teacher how you knew that God answered your prayers. It seemed to me, I said, that if God gave people what they wanted, they said He answered their prayers, but if God didn't give them what they wanted, people still said He listened to their prayers. What would God have to do, I asked, to convince people He wasn't interested? She turned to the class and said, "And now we'll all pray for Anna," and they did.

But I had a checkered past even then and should have appreciated my ability to offend. My first memory is of turning a piano stool on its side and hiding behind it with a collection of empty glass milk bottles. When someone walked by, I would pop up and throw a glass milk bottle at them, then duck back down. It didn't end well. Fortunately, those diapers absorbed some of the walloping that followed.

My next memory isn't a memory at all, but a story my kindergarten teacher told me when I was grown. She told all of the five-year-olds to rest by putting their feet on the floor, their hands on their desks and their heads on their hands. She said I did all of it, then raised my head, looked straight at her, and lifted one foot.

All I can remember of first grade is that the penalty for talking too much was being paddled behind the screen that held our coats. I spent a lot of first grade behind the screen. In fourth grade, I got straight As except for a D in conduct. I lived for recess. Once my older sister came to my fourth grade classroom door with a message for me. When the door was opened, she saw that all the other girls were wearing skirts and not the jeans I had vehemently insisted to my mother that they were wearing. In fact, I was the only girl in jeans in that North Carolina classroom in 1956. Unfortunately, the snitch went home and told my mother. I thought the deception justified: How can you wear a skirt when you had your own gang at recess chasing other gangs through the woods? We called it a gang, not knowing any better, although all we did essentially was play tag. Thank God all that was way back then. Today someone would have diagnosed me as ADHD and stuffed Ritalin down my throat.

By fifth grade I was playing tight end on the football team at recess with the boys. Anyone could join, but the other girls were all sitting on the rocks, combing their hair and talking. I could not fathom that. Class was for talking; recess was for playing. A few years ago, I went to a class reunion and talked with my best girlfriends from that era. Forty years later they wanted to know what on earth I was doing running around the woods with a stick, and I wanted to know how they could just sit on those rocks and talk.

In the summer between fifth and sixth grade, I put a basketball in the basket on the front of my bike and pedaled a few miles to our school's aging high school gym. The doors were locked so I went around to the back and found a boarded-up broken window. I pulled the boards off, threw the basketball in, and climbed after it. I discovered heaven: the sheer silence of the cavernous place, the sound of a single ball dribbling, the smell of the leather ball, the light from the high windows shapeshifting on the floor through the dust, and the chance to play and play and play. Of course, there was the small matter of the heat in a boarded-up building in the North Carolina summer. But I was a Southern girl, and heat could be ignored. The silence was broken only by the sound of the ball swooshing through the net or banging off the boards. The peace of that space was worth ignoring the heat. After that, I fled the house almost every summer day and shot baskets for, literally, all day in the old, boarded-up gym, a practice I continued through high school. I developed a rhythm. Each time I started shooting close to the basket, moving all around it, and then worked systematically away. I worked on a "boy's" jump

Chapter 2. Beginnings

shot—releasing the ball at the top of the jump, but I was never strong enough to do that shot from very far.

One day I was working on the left hook I didn't really master until I pulled a ligament in my right hand and had no other way to shoot. I didn't hear the gym doors opening. I stopped short when the girls' high school coach walked in. I didn't know the term "breaking and entering" then, but I knew I had no permission to be there and that I had pulled a board off to get in. He asked me how I got in. I told him I crawled through a back window, neglecting to mention the board I had plied off. He just looked at me, and I could smell cooked goose. But after that, he opened the gym for me every day in the summer. The breeze from the open doors just enhanced heaven. The boys came to play off and on, never the girls. I was the only one who stayed all day. I played with the high school boys, and once when I was in high school, they took me across the bridge to play when they informally faced their archrivals, the next town over. My routine of practicing became almost invariant: three hours or more after school during the year shooting at my rickety basket at home, even on days we had practice after school, and all day in the gym in the summer.

If you practice that much you will eventually get good, especially when the other girls are only showing up for official practice during the season. I started every game my freshman year, but I also fouled out of every game. You can't block out under the boards with high school boys and adjust easily to the no-touch game of girls' basketball in the early '60s. I averaged 26 points a game my sophomore year with a high of 44 one night when the basket seemed four feet wide. Those numbers led to consequences. My last two years I never played a game without being double-teamed. And some teams took it further. One night the first time I shot a girl slapped me, knocking out a contact lens. After that, every time I shot, a girl hit me. The opposing team fouled out five guards that night, and I went to the line 25 times. It wasn't a great strategy. I wasn't that bad at free throws. The double-teaming was more effective. I was no Larry Bird and my high scoring ended. Not to mention my beloved coach ran away with an all-state guard in the middle of my junior year, and the team never recovered.[1] Basketball had become my life, and abandonment decentered me. The new coach was not a great coach and made a poor contrast with the original coach who, I have been told, never had a losing season with any sport he coached. Certainly, he was the best coach I ever had in anything. With the tunnel vision that athletes have, I could not understand how marrying Freida was more important that chasing the conference championship.

I did get an offer the summer after high school to play on a women's pro team. Women's pro teams back then played comedy routines, much like the Harlem Globetrotters; there was no women's pro league. They were called the Redheads or the Hazel Walkers or some such. Lord, were those comedy women good! I once saw the Hazel Walkers take apart a male Marine team with a 6'8" center when the play got serious for a few minutes. I gave my father the letter inviting me to join a pro team for a European tour. He read the handwritten note filled with misspellings and poor grammar. He looked up. "Honey," he said, "you're going to college." And that was that.

There was no women's basketball program at Wake Forest or the University of North Carolina between 1964 and 1968 when I attended. Most colleges didn't have them in those days. There was still pick-up ball, 30 years of it playing with men after that, and those experiences were closer to the days in the cavernous, silent gym than games filled with spectators ever could have been. Playing for the love of it. Playing because you are completely in the moment. Playing because afterward the neurons were all scrubbed clean. Playing with whoever shows up at whatever level they are. Playing because you know men in a different way when you play ball with them. You are sports buddies, one of the group, and you realize—or at least I did in high school—just how strangely they treat most girls. High school boys never treated girls like buddies back then, but only as potential sex partners. I'm not sure they knew we were human.

In the fifties and early sixties in the South, stereotypes were

Chapter 2. Beginnings

Platonic forms covered in cement, and they governed how you talked and what you said, how you dressed, and who you could be. You had better fit into one of those stereotypes or no one knew what to do with you. You were an outcast. The problem was, there was only one stereotype for a girl then, and it was "Southern Lady." Unfortunately, Southern Lady and I were never on speaking terms. Our issues went beyond my love of sports and intolerance of inactivity.

Every year for Christmas when I was little, my parents gave me a new doll, and every year I beat up my two-year-younger brother and took his cars and trucks. I didn't want the stupid doll. By elementary school my most treasured possessions were a bike and a basketball, and I lived in dread of getting dressed up for Easter Sunday. My brother asked me as an adult if I knew how many kids were afraid to come into our yard, and I didn't. I don't remember myself as violent, maybe just a little feisty. I asked him once if I was actually violent as a child. "No," he said kindly, and then added "just aggressive. All anyone had to do was look at how you played basketball to see you meant business. You would take out someone to get to the basket." He once told me as a child he was locked in a shack he and some friends had built in the swamp when the shack was set on fire by some neighborhood bullies. He somehow managed to break out. He didn't tell me at the time, he said, because he was afraid of what I would do to them. He also reminded me that when he was little and people picked on him, he went and got me. "By talking or by other means," he said, "you made it clear they should not be saying those things."

Two years older, I was bigger and stronger than my brother up until adolescence, and I won most of our early fights. I also had better acting skills, and he got blamed for starting most of the fights. Once he swung at me and missed and broke his hand. Of course, adolescence ended that. When I was 14 and he was 12, my days of superior strength were over. With wit born of desperation, I switched to verbal taunting and claimed that physical fighting was for babies. But that Christmas he was given boxing gloves and my family, tired of all those years of my picking on him, egged on the fight he wanted.

Pride made me agree, but luck got me through. He swung, I ducked, landed a lucky punch and that was it: my last fight and I went out on top. Southern Lady was nowhere in sight.

If this makes it sound like my brother was a victim, it was not for long. When he got his adolescent growth spurt, he became tougher than me. It's hard to play center on a high school football team at 150 pounds but he did. Once he played most of a game with broken ribs. My parents didn't know they were broken until later that night when they found him crawling up the stairs.

My father was a country doc, and he encouraged toughness. He had once broken his finger in a baseball game as a high school student. With the bone sticking out, he went over to a teammate and asked him to put the bone back in—no doubt just to see his friend's nauseous face as the friend sat down on the field. I broke my nose a couple of times in basketball games. My father would come down to the court, straighten it out using a fountain pen as a guide, and send me back into the game. Was that sane? Am I endorsing it? Of course not. But he did it.

I was able to duck most of adolescence hiding in the gym, but not all of it. Clueless socially, I had a best friend who was everything I wasn't. Poised and graceful Jennie knew how to say the right thing, do the right thing, and dress the right way. On my side I had a decent jump shot, was hell under the boards, and loved to slalom water ski.

My issues with Southern Lady came to a head in my teen years. If no one in my tiny high school knew what to make of a girl who didn't like girl things and loved sports, the one who had the least clue was me. I got called "dyke" now and then because any girl who played sports was so branded. I began to wonder if I was gay. That would at least have been an identity, although a problematic one in 1960 in a small town in the South. The real problem for me with being gay was boys. They were so delicious looking. They smelled right, and they felt right when you put your arms around them. I had my first boyfriend in fifth grade, and we rode our bikes all over town, attending 15-cent movies and picnicking in the woods. I had a boyfriend during

Chapter 2. Beginnings

my freshman year in high school, a sweet, smiling, good-natured boy who later became a fighter pilot. Later I had another one who was not so sweet and tried to strangle me one night, although half-heartedly. He became a dentist. I had a third who moved away to a much larger school. The boys' basketball team he had been on in my hometown had won the state championship in their division three years in a row and had won 91 consecutive games along the way. One night I drove 90 miles to see him play basketball at his new, much larger school in a bigger division. He was a good player and was in the starting line-up at this much bigger school. He had to guard a tall, skinny kid that night, and just looking at the kid, I thought Jeffrey could take him. It was not to be. The tall, skinny kid scored 42 points that night and made Jeffrey look like he was planted on the court. Dazed afterward, I asked, "Who the heck was that?"

"Oh," I was told. "He's a big high school star out of Raleigh. His name is Pete Maravich."[2]

I liked boys. I liked them as sports buddies, and I liked them as boyfriends. I liked making out with them. Sex was out. Actually having sex with a boy would have branded you a whore in the South in those days and that stereotype was fatal. Still, I liked the thought of sex with a boy, and I thought about it a lot. I didn't feel much of anything towards girls except that most seemed to live in a world that bored me into a coma. Being gay wasn't going to work out.

But if I wasn't gay, who was I? I didn't know any girls like me. I didn't know of any athletes who were women at that time. I thought I was a freak. I certainly wasn't like my mother who was hysterical most of the time and never thought the sun should set on a day she didn't scream at somebody. I identified with my father, who was far more logical and even-tempered than she. But identifying with males only went so far. I liked my girl's body. It felt like me, like I belonged in it. I never had a desire to trade it in.

And so adolescence went. I didn't know what the heck I was. There were categories and I didn't seem to fit in any of them. In this day and time, post–Title IX, with female athletes as plentiful and admired as male, it is difficult to appreciate just how isolated and pained a fanatical female gym rat could feel growing up in the '50s and early '60s in a small town in the South.

And then came Billy Jean King. It was too late to save me from my adolescent angst but welcome all the same. I saw her on TV playing a tennis match and she changed everything. Here was a woman who played with a ferocity and intensity I understood. I looked at the faces of other women tennis players and, for the first time, saw my own. They were ferocious competitors. They practiced relentlessly. They would take your head off with a serve. They didn't feel one bit sorry when they won, and they did not apologize for the hard work they put in. Some were straight; some were gay. It didn't matter. They were athletes and they were women. None of them were on good terms with Southern Lady.

For the record, I don't want to be Bill Russell anymore when I grow up. I want to be Larry Bird, but I have to face it now: the Celtics, it seems, missed their opportunity to draft me. I have a Ph.D. from Harvard and there have been awards along the way now and then and compliments as well. But the greatest compliment I ever received was from the boys' basketball coach in our town. He was a legend in small-town Class A basketball, a man whose teams at Beaufort High won three state championships in a row and 91 consecutive games—still a North Carolina high school record. In his last state championship, he told the *Raleigh News & Observer* that his best player was on the bench and spoke of the gym rat who thought she was a freak.

Chapter 3

On Malice

I am a long way from a gym. I am a grown-up now—or pass as one—and I am in court again, trying this time to keep an 18-year-old man in prison for as long as the law will allow—preferably his entire life. Generally, I believe in rehabilitation, but I draw the line at men who abduct and murder children. His first try at abduction and murder was an adult jogger who fought him off. Actually, he is suspected of assaulting two joggers, but there is DNA evidence to conclusively prove he was the offender in only one of the cases. The second jogger didn't see him and there was no DNA so he wasn't charged. When he was unsuccessful with the adults, he decided he needed to find someone smaller and weaker.

I am on the stand, watching him as I testify. You might think geek; you surely wouldn't think "half-pipe" or "football." Dark-haired, pudgy, a certain intensity in the eyes, he is staring at me from a distance of about eight feet while I testify. I have the distinct impression he would take my throat out with a spoon if he could. He has a habit of fantasizing about such things—and acting on them. I had only seen that look once before while testifying, but it is unforgettable, and the pure malevolence is likely what the victim saw as well.

He is a sadist, likely a necrophiliac, the killer of a 10-year-old girl who caught his eye somewhere before he waited for her at a blind spot on the street where she walked to elementary school. There are four defense attorneys sitting next to him. The two men are farthest from him, sitting straight up, hands folded on the table in front of them and staring straight ahead. Their body language says they have no connection to the man at the end of the table, and if God could just pick them up and drop them in the middle of the Atlantic Ocean, they would appreciate it.

Not so for the two female attorneys. The one responsible for crossing me is playing Jack-in-the-box while I testify on direct. She pops up and down with endless objections to my testimony. They are not compelling, and she loses most of them, but they are curiously emotional. Finally, she pops up and says, "Your honor, I am overwhelmed. I am speechless." Later I learn that the prosecutor was thinking what I and many of the spectators were: would that it were so. I find myself wondering what kind of legal objection "speechless" is.

After I testify, I notice her leaning close to the defendant and rubbing his back. Her gesture is maternal—poor child who just made a mistake. It is also strangely obscene under the circumstances. I am used to offenders who suck people in, but this signifies a lack of reality testing on her part. The "poor child" masturbated to porn of children being dismembered as a warm-up. He abducted, raped, and strangled a child, before finally putting her face down in scalding water to make sure she was dead. He then dismembered her, cutting out each organ carefully and identifying it before flushing it down the toilet. He kept the head and several body parts under the house. The rest of the child he tossed into a plastic bag and left in another part of town to mislead police. He used chloroform on one of the female joggers he attacked. Both of them fought him off. He had picked out a place to drop the body of one of them before the attack. Does the female defense attorney know what he'd do to her if he got the chance?

The defendant's mother has a better grasp of reality. She has been there for every court hearing, and she wore purple every time, the favorite color of the victim. With a choice of color, she said over and over again, "I love my son still, but I am horrified by what he did." Her, I understand.

His name is Austin Sigg[1] and police had taken his DNA after a neighbor called in a tip following an Amber alert, thinking it strange

Chapter 3. On Malice

that a teenager would drop out of high school to become a mortician. The DNA results weren't back yet, but Sigg knew what they would be. His mom had just gotten back from work when Austin told her. She sobbed and asked why and where and how—and learned there were body parts hidden under her home. She asked him if he wanted to call the police or wanted her to. It doesn't appear she considered any other option. It is less clear to me that he expected that. Did he think she might "help" in some other way: a car, a ticket to another country? Once before, she had caught him with child porn and had not called the police but put him into treatment instead. But if it were possible for her to underestimate the extent of his sexual interest in young children, it was not possible to underestimate this. When on the phone with 911, she suddenly said, "I can't breathe." And what mother could have?

I am testifying at the sentencing. Colorado law says an offender who was under 18 at the time of the offense cannot be sentenced to life without parole for any one charge. Sigg was three months shy of his 18th birthday at the time of the killing, even younger when he tried to chloroform and abduct the jogger he is charged with. The prosecutor wants the sentences consecutive, which would keep him in forever. The defense, of course, does not and hence the contested hearing.

I have read 10,000 pages of records and have written a lengthy report on types of offenders and what kind he is, on why this wasn't an "adolescent" offense, mitigated by the developmental immaturity of the adolescent brain, on the reasons for the killing or lack thereof: Sigg was neither abused nor bullied nor mentally ill. But on the stand, I wonder as I sometimes do—did I really get a Ph.D. to be able to say that a man who would abduct, rape, torture, kill, and dismember a 10-year-old girl is dangerous? Let's take the first 100 people who walk by on the street and ask them. Who besides the pop-up, Jack-in-the-box lawyer would think otherwise?

But there is a more pressing issue for me: how do I get across to the judge what I think without putting worse pictures in the minds of the family. There are issues surrounding the girl's death. Sigg is a self-serving reporter, and while it is impossible to paint a good picture of dismembering a child, he has painted an image of a very quick death with nothing but letting her watch Netflix preceding it. It is most certainly not true, but do I need to say that? And how specific do I have to be? These people—the family and friends, the girl's mother with the dark pits for eyes, the police who searched for the child, the stunned community members who are here—they all have to live with the pictures in their heads. Do I need to add to them?

Yes, I know. People think of expert witnesses as court whores who say whatever they are paid to say. But while we have more than our share, being a court whore is not actually a necessary condition for testifying in court. For those who aren't, the issues are different than most people think. Today this is my issue. I say what is wrong with Sigg's account, why I think it is incomplete. I allude to other possibilities, but I am vague. I do not say everything that I think. I can afford not to. In the middle of my testimony the judge waves off objections to questions about recidivism, saying, "I'm not worried about recidivism," and we all relax. He isn't going to let him out. That is, we relax as much as you can relax when you are in the presence of malevolence.

I will wait until after the appeals are over, and then I will see if he will talk to me. Today he would not, but prison is boring, and many offenders are narcissists who want to brag about how clever they are, even after being caught. And this is what I do. I talk to men like this in prison and in civil commitment centers and try to understand how they think and what they feel. I'll be sitting in that chair again. When I am, I want to lay absolutely accurate information on the table. The iconic image of justice is of a statuesque female wearing a blindfold and holding up a scale. Blind justice is not actually that good an idea. Blind to race, ethnicity, standing in the community, socio-economic status, yes, but blind about the motivations and risk posed by an offender, not so good.

Violence doesn't make sense, not to most of us. That's under-

Chapter 3. On Malice

standable and good for one's peace of mind. Life is easier if you don't spend your days trying to make sense of horrible acts. There are motivations we can all relate to and motivations we can't. Ironically, we know what pedophiles feel—sexual attraction. We know desire and can shudder at the thought of feeling it for young children. But there are motivations outside the normal range that have no echo in most human beings, just as there are sounds that humans can't hear and other animals can. We are not going to find those motivations in ourselves and empathize with others who have them. The high that one offender gets from strangling a child will find no resonance in us.

The problem comes when we try to "make pretty," to change disagreeable and frightening motivations to something we can empathize with and fear less. When "nice" people are faced with motivations they do not understand and cannot feel empathy for, they distort the motivations into something they can relate to. A child with extensive cigarette burns is described by an evaluator as a victim of an overwhelmed parent who "lost it." Cigarette burns are never a result of sudden, overwhelming anger. A backhand or even a broken arm can be, but cigarette burns over a period of time are a product of someone who is very much in control of themselves and wants to deliberately inflict pain. Inflicting pain for the high it gives the offender turns, in the hands of a naïve evaluator, into a watered-down version of itself. It is labelled a "loss of control," a "failure to understand boundaries," a "lack of parenting skills." Put the offender in a parenting class; he'll be fine. After the parenting class, the reunification can begin. Such an evaluator simply can't believe that malice exists. Failure to recognize violent cognitions and motivations for what they are results in underestimating the risk such offenders pose.

"Let the healing begin," one defense attorney said, in a case where a child was starved, forced to sleep in a cabinet under the sink every night that was so tight that she had a permanent scar on one shoulder where a piece of metal protruded into her back. Although she was starving, she kept a long red coat on at school, and the teachers never knew. The case was only discovered when a brother broke most of the bones in her hands. At that point one of her teachers said, "We wondered why she had those red marks on her face from her ear to her mouth." They were, of course, gag marks. The defense attorney wanted to start the reunification process immediately. Fortunately, the judge disagreed.

One of the most popular theories for treating sex offenders today, the Good Lives Model, assumes that everyone has the same basic needs and wants the same things out of life. It's just that offenders don't know how to get them in "socially acceptable" ways. If treatment helps them to meet their needs in better ways, the theory goes, they will stop offending. This is actually true of many low-risk offenders. But Jerry Sandusky had a good life. He certainly had access to adult women. He just preferred children. Likewise, Ted Bundy had all the skills he needed to be successful, but the thrill he got from abduction and murder was far greater than what he got by going to law school and having consensual sex with willing partners.

Thomas Sowell, the American economist and political philosopher, wrote, "One of the common failings among honorable people is a failure to appreciate how thoroughly dishonorable some other people can be, and how dangerous it is to trust them." It is difficult for most people, and impossible for some, to recognize malevolence. Of course, no one—well, almost no one—can miss the malice in Sigg, which is why the sea of spectators at the trial looked as though they had taken LSD and were on a nightmarish trip. But there are plenty of other occasions where dangerous men and women are put on the street because someone buys "sorry."

Why can I and others see malice when some cannot no matter how egregious the crimes? I cannot speak for others, but I know why I can see it. I had a head start. I had a personality disordered mother who was more cruel than crazy. Malice was a steady breeze blowing through my childhood. The type I lived with was not the sort of big-time malice that results in blood on the floor or trips to the hospital, but it was kin.

Chapter 4

Nemesis

When I was four years old my mother's favorite lines to me were "You think you're something special. You think you're a queen bee. You're nothing but a snake in the grass." I don't know how early she started saying that. I can remember the comments and their frequency from age four. The litany continued throughout my childhood. There were beatings, of course, along with the emotional abuse. Corporal punishment was common in the South in the '50s but my mother's discipline was more extreme and for different reasons than most parents. Spill a glass of milk as a preschooler, and the slap in the face was immediate. The slaps in the face would leave a red imprint of the entire hand. Bother her, make too much noise, stay up too late reading—the switch left marks that could be seen a day later. You weren't hit for reading during the day, but you were told, "You always have your nose in a book." The beatings were not the kinds of injuries that would send you to the hospital; the emotional abuse cut deeper. The jokes she made cut to the bone. She and my father, she liked to say, had stayed married because they agreed whoever asked for a divorce had to take the kids. Ha, ha, ha. No matter how many times she said it, she thought it funny. Even as young children we got the point. She also said on many occasions she didn't want any of her children living within 1,000 miles of her when we grew up. Early on, I came to agree.

A few years ago, my best friend from childhood asked me if I remembered the day she and I were riding in a car with my mother. My friend and I were in the back seat, and I asked my mother a question. She didn't answer. I didn't think she heard me and asked again.

Again, she didn't answer. I spoke up once more and suddenly my mother screamed, "Do I have to hit you to shut you up?" It scared my friend out of her skin, and 50 years later she still remembered it. I just laughed when she told me. Of course, I didn't remember. That could have been any day in my childhood.

My biggest crime was being my father's favorite child. There were three of us then, but my older sister was never in the running. My father was called into the service shortly after her birth, and my parents left the baby with my grandparents for a year while my mother followed my father from base to base until he was deployed to England. My mother came back to reclaim her in a year while my father went to war, but even when he returned, neither parent doted on her. The parent/child bonding never recovered for either parent and Linda became the lost, left-out child. Brighter and more loving than any of us, she was pudgy as a child, had bad acne as an adolescent, and was never an athlete. These things did not endear her, especially to my mother.

My brother was a more likely candidate but had a strange love-hate relationship with my mother I didn't understand until I was much older. Why my father didn't dote on him as he did me, I've never known, but I was the yellow-haired joy of my father's life, the "apple of his eye," hence earning my mother's ever-lasting enmity. She was a formidable opponent.

Even so, there was a gift in the consistency of the enmity. My mother was an enemy soldier through and through. I learned early on she was never there for me. She was not alternately warm and scathing as she was with my brother or simply distant and uninterested as she was with my sister. Neither seemed a threat to her. No doubt the psychoanalysts would have a field day, but I didn't know psychoanalytic theory at age four. All I knew was that she was mean to me pretty much all the time and didn't like to be touched. Because she was so consistently hurtful, I never really bonded with her, and years later that would set me free.

When my first child was small, I remember once having lunch

Chapter 4. Nemesis

with my mother and a genuine Southern Lady, a warm and loving, soft-spoken woman who was a friend my mother had not yet alienated. My mother, for God knows what reasons, decided to tell a tale she thought funny of my brother's first grade teacher sending a note home from school. "Please help him remember to bring a pencil to school," it said. "He keeps forgetting." The note infuriated my mother. She took it that my brother was making the school think they couldn't afford to buy him pencils. "I called him in real sweet," she said, "and then when he got close, I got a hold of him and beat the living hell out of him." Our lunch companion nearly choked. "We never beat our children ..." she said tentatively. I ignored her. All I could see was my brother's trusting face as he ran to my mother. I looked at my mother and said, "You better never lay a hand on one of mine."

"That's your choice," she said, bowing to my authority as their mother, but at the same time justifying her right to choose how she treated us. Still, I never really trusted her around my children when they were young and was always hovering when she was there.

While my mother's hatred of me was unrelenting, by contrast, she was alternately loving and raging toward my brother with no warning when she would switch. He was her favorite when she was in a good mood, but over and over she sucked him in, only to scream at or beat or otherwise abuse him. She made him walk to her knowing he'd be slapped. She made him put his hands down and she'd tell him which side of his face she was going to hit. Then she would slap him as hard as she could. Then she would do it again. This would go on for a while. Sometimes she made him cut the switch she beat him with. At other times, she stroked his forehead and told him she loved him. My brother eventually put an end to the physical abuse. All in all, though, he got a far worse deal than I. Because she went back and forth, he came to love and hate her. He did not go down to see her for the last 12 years of her life, although he called her every Sunday night.

She never really made any attempt to suck me in. The battle lines were drawn by four. As a result, I wouldn't get the switch she'd beat me with. I wouldn't walk up to her to be slapped. When she wanted to beat me, she had to catch me. I ran, slamming the screen door behind me. At 12 I quit calling her "Mother" and called her Kate[1] instead. I spent my teenage years in the gym.

Over and over my father begged me to try to get along with my mother, by which he meant don't do anything to upset her. Neither my brother nor I knew why, but he loved her. None of us were trying to upset my mother. It's just that volcanoes don't care who's walking by. When something irritated my mother—and anything could irritate her—she exploded and tried her best to transfer that effect to the nearest living creature. She was a sieve for negative affect, incapable of containing it. It went right through her, passed along to the next available host. Once that person was in tears my mother felt much better. The reader will no doubt conclude there was something wrong with her—perhaps there were traumas in her background of which I knew nothing. Perhaps there were, but as someone raised by a narcissistic and possibly borderline mother, I decided early on that "mental illness is no excuse for bad manners." In the name of their own pain, there are people who will eat you alive, and they are just as dangerous as the people who do it for sport. "Live or die," Anne Sexton wrote, "but don't poison everything." Can't we all just agree on that, at least?

Early on I decided I did not want to be my mother. In many ways this defined my childhood and probably much of my life. If my mother was overweight and complained about it constantly, I would be forever lean. If my mother made everyone wait on her, bring her food and drink and whatever else she wanted, I would be relentlessly self-sufficient. If my mother wanted nothing more than to sit and watch TV, I would spend my life in the gym. To this day I don't own a TV. When my mother said she "didn't like to learn new things," she sent me on a life-long journey of learning and exploration. If my mother only read the *Reader's Digest* version of books, I would read unabridged versions incessantly. If my mother was labile and

Chapter 4. Nemesis

illogical, I would fall in love with logic and with calm. Pick your nemesis carefully. She will define you.

Research for decades has shown that if a child has one adult who cares for them and believes in them, either inside or outside the home, they can make it through adverse circumstances. The Center on the Developing Child at Harvard, for example, wrote in a 2022 webpage on resilience in children, "The single most common factor for children who develop resilience is at least one stable and committed relationship with a supportive parent, caregiver, or other adult" (https://developingchild.harvard.edu/science/key-concepts/resilience/). I had one, my father, and I had the genetics of North Carolina fishermen and women who plied their trade by facing the treacherous Atlantic over and over in all kinds of weather. I take no credit for surviving my mother. It was my father who lit the spark long ago and no doubt the "luck of the genetic draw" that helped me survive.

When friends start talking about difficult mothers, I can hold my own in most company. Of course, I can't hold my own everywhere. My mother never locked me in the basement for five years or broke every bone in my hands or did some of the things I've seen in cases I have had, but I have a contender in most groups. Once a boyfriend came home with me as an adult and said to me that despite my descriptions of her, she seemed like a nice old lady. I asked him if I had told him about the time she cultivated her relationship with a rich older woman and persuaded her to put my mother in her will as the sole inheritor of her estate instead of the woman's children. I actually screamed at my mother for that but to no avail.

I needn't have bothered. Once the old lady signed the will, my mother backed off, thinking the deed was done. Fortunately, the lady changed her will and left everything to someone my mother called "a con man" who lived in town. My mother was furious when she found out. Perhaps he wasn't a con man or perhaps the lady changed her mind again, because my sister assures me the estate eventually was left with a neighbor who was not a con man and had helped the woman a great deal.

When the old lady died, someone from the estate called asking if my mother knew where she might have put a valuable coin collection she had owned. My mother told him she had no idea. I found out later it was in a safe in my mother's bedroom. I told my mother it was immoral and *illegal* to keep the coin collection. Another screaming match. My mother said she deserved the coins for all the things she had done for the older woman, who had ungratefully turned around and changed her will. I kept trying to explain the meaning of "grand theft" to her but was met with "You don't know what you're talking about." She sent the coins to my brother to sell as I would have nothing to do with them. As a lawyer, he did not consider fencing stolen goods an option. He told her he was trying but couldn't find a buyer. He stalled and eventually sent the coins back. Should I have called the police and turned in my 80-year-old mother? I didn't. I didn't have the heart to send an 80-year-old to jail and no proof of anything besides. She could simply have said the old lady gave them to her. Too, in that small town, where my father was a local legend, I don't believe there was any chance she would have even been investigated. I'm sure friends and relatives of the old lady would think I should have tried.

My elder sister was killed in a parachuting accident when I was 19 and she was 24. I learned then that although my mother was a narcissist and could be unfathomably cruel, there were nonetheless limits. She genuinely grieved my sister's death, and by all accounts, she changed her parenting after my sister died. Another sister, younger than I am by 10 years, describes a very different childhood from the one I had. When I sent an early draft of this memoir to her, she responded that she had a very different experience with Kate for most of her childhood. Of course, most of it occurred after my sister died. My mother changed to the point she was no longer cruel to young children. Her daughter, my niece, told me recently that my mother never laid a hand on her and was her favorite grandmother. It made me smile. Change matters, and it was the first time in my life that I had been proud of my mother.

It was too late for my mother and me, and our relationship was

Chapter 4. Nemesis

never redeemed. I was not there to see my mother's behavior toward my younger sibling, and she retained enough of the old Kate to keep our phone conversations short. I found to my surprise that after I moved away my anger and my hatred died down. You have to be attached to someone to really hate them, and I just was never that attached to her. People don't get attached to enemy soldiers, only to spies. It was a relief not to carry her around anymore, to let her go.

What was harder for me was the realization as an adult that my beloved father could have protected us but didn't. As a child, I had them figured out: he was the good parent, the one who lit up when we came running into his arms when he came home from work. She was the bad parent, the one who didn't like to be touched and who could explode at any time. I wasn't a dumb kid, but I never managed to see how he colluded with her treatment of us. As a young doctor, he had landed in Normandy in the second wave and stitched up soldiers so close to the fighting in Czechoslovakia that bullets flew through the tents and patients begged the doctors to get down. Still, he couldn't stand up to her. My father did not protect us and could have. It was a bitter realization.

With the detachment from my mother came a kind of peace. I called every few months after my father died, just to make sure she was OK. He would have wanted me to. But I no longer wanted her to get hit by a bus. I even hoped things went well for her. We had a kind of truce.

The truce was broken once, though, when my father was dying, and at that time I came close to killing her. My father collapsed one day in his late seventies, whether by heart attack or stroke we never knew. He was in the bathroom when a young grandson came running in to tell my mother he was slumped on the floor against the wall. My mother, with no less than 30 years of warning that my father might have another heart attack, had never learned CPR. She called the ambulance and some neighbors but did nothing else. When they arrived almost 10 minutes later, he could not be revived and never regained consciousness.

She called to tell me, and when I said I would fly down immediately, she said not to come, she would need us more later. She could not fathom that his children might want to say goodbye to him. I didn't bother arguing. I hung up the phone and made reservations. When I arrived at the ICU (which was named for him),[2] I asked her to give me a few minutes alone with him; there were things I wanted to say. I had thought about it going down and it seemed to me that dying was a scary business and, knowing my father, he would be most worried about leaving his children. Who knew if an unconscious mind could hear, but I didn't know it couldn't, and I wanted to do whatever I could to ease his passing. By then I had been told he would not recover.

When my mother left the room, I told my father that it would be wonderful if he could stay, but that if he couldn't, then not to worry about us. He had been a great father. He had been a great doctor. All of his children were grown and independent. We were all going to be fine. I went on in this vein for some time, and felt, at least, I had done what I could to make his passing peaceful.

When I told my mother it was OK to come in, she walked in, sat down heavily, and said in a loud voice, "Well, I guess I'll just starve to death." My mother was living on a large waterfront property across from an uninhabited island where banker ponies run wild. The property was worth close to a million dollars. She wasn't going to starve to death. She then went on about her beach club membership, hinting I should pay her dues for her. I should have had warning she was capable of this. When my father had his first heart surgery, which carried an 18 percent chance of dying on the table, my mother took all of us aback by exploding in the motel room the night before: "What about me? You are all young. You have your families. But what about me?" Everything was always about my mother.

But that day in the ICU, while I was trying to make my father's passing easier, my mother's words caught me completely unaware. I knew my father was devastated if he heard them. She had just undone all I had tried to do. Even his dying wasn't about him; it was once again about her. For the one and only time in my life I was flooded

Chapter 4. Nemesis

with an urge to kill someone so intense I didn't think I could control it. The first thing that flashed through my mind was an image of a gun, the steel grip almost blue in my mind's eye. Luckily, I had no gun. Next, I thought, "If I get my hands around her scrawny neck, there aren't enough staff on this floor to pry them off. There may not be enough in this hospital." I started shaking slightly with the intensity of the rage. Then I found the thought, "You can't kill your mother while your father is on his deathbed; it would upset him greatly." "Upset him greatly" sounds stilted as I write it now, but at the time it was, literally, a lifesaver. I looked at the door, thinking if I could just get out of the room, I would be OK. I slowly got up and started walking to the door repeating to myself, "You can't kill her while he's on his death bed; it will upset…. You can't kill her…." I didn't look at her. I knew if I did, the thought might not be enough to stop me. She continued to jabber about her fantasy money problems and her desire to keep her beach club membership.

I got myself out of the room and to a phone. I called a friend and got her voice mail. "I'm going to kill her," I said. "I am absolutely going to kill her. I'm afraid to go back in there because I will kill her." I went on regurgitating the rage into the phone. Other family arrived shortly after that, and the tide turned on the urge, and it slowly receded.

Except for my father's funeral, I had not been back home for a decade when my mother herself died years later although I called regularly. My brother and I both came down when she was dying. My brother had an attack of appendicitis on the plane so severe he was taken to the hospital immediately for surgery on his arrival. Who knows if the stress of going down there after 20 to 30 years played a role? When I walked into my mother's room, Kate looked at me and started to speak. I leaned over to hear her say, "You're just here because I'm dying."

"That's true," I said. "I'm here because you're dying." I left out the "just" but we both knew it was there. My mother and I, oddly enough, didn't lie to each other. It was the only thing she said to me.

She had decided it was time to go and was refusing food or any kind of feeding tube. She lapsed into a coma, and we realized we didn't know what she wanted us to do about liquids. The nurses kept putting IVs in and she kept pulling them out. Did she mean she didn't want them, or was she just delirious? We wanted to at least keep her comfortable. While we debated, a nurse came in to re-insert the IV, and my mother roused herself from her coma and grabbed the nurse's arm. "What about 'no' don't you understand?" she said and sank back into unconsciousness. I always thought my mother lived a long life because even God didn't want to take on my mother.

By the time she died, my mother had few friends left, having alienated most of them over the years. A few came to her funeral; most former friends didn't. My mother and my father both had numerous relatives Down East, only 20 miles away. When my father died, the church was filled with relatives from both sides. Very few relatives of either side came to my mother's funeral. Very few. Some of my family members were hurt by this. I understood completely.

My father was right that I could have been more willing to compromise as a child than I was, but it would have done little good. My mother was not the compromising type. At that time in her life, it was battle or be beaten down, and my mother never played fair. Is it any wonder that I loved sports? Any wonder I found the silence of an empty gym alluring and played all day by myself? Sports had rules that didn't change in the middle of the game. Sports were a meritocracy. You made the basket, and they counted the points. Sports were logical, and they were designed to be fair.

Our weaknesses are our strengths and our strengths our weaknesses, depending on the context. The expert witnesses I have seen fold on the stand and agree with things they know aren't true can't stand disagreeing with the opposing attorney. They want him or her to like them. They want the social fabric between them to lay smooth and unruffled. But I don't come from the land of smooth and unruffled social fabric stretching between people. I come from the land of trench warfare and, as a result, I am just not that easy to push.

Chapter 4. Nemesis

I quite literally spent my childhood fighting with my mother. Playing pick-up ball for 30 years and going under the boards with men who were bigger and stronger than I was a piece of cake compared to Kate. It's true also that I have found court a setting where the ability to battle was an asset. Still, I won't pretend there wasn't a price to pay. By age 16 I was driving 125 miles an hour on North Carolina back country roads and wondering, with some detachment, whether the car would make the next curve or not. No question my mother got to me. If I survived and finally let go of my anger, it was because I wore enough armor in my childhood to make a medieval knight proud. "Every form of refuge has its price," Don Henley and Glenn Fry wrote. Wear armor too long and it will stick to your skin: it is nearly impossible to remove when you don't need it anymore. After two failed marriages I have figured out I am probably not the easiest person to live with. What most people start out with, the ability to be a nice, relaxed person around other people, has taken me a lifetime to learn. For many years, I had a wariness around people, especially groups, that approached paranoia. On some level I was always expecting attack. Even today I recharge my batteries in solitude. Thomas Keating wrote, "God's first language is Silence. Everything else is a translation." It is ironic that I have lived such a public life while finding more peace in solitude than anywhere else.

Still, I don't want to exaggerate and leave the reader with the impression that I am a hermit living in a cave. I may need time alone and cherish nature and animals, but I have been fortunate to be able to maintain close friends all my life. I met two of my best friends when we were four years old. One died recently and on her deathbed said to me that we had been "best friends all our lives." My other best friend is a Toronto urbanite who takes her nature on the Discovery Channel. We talk almost every day and have for over two decades. For the past 30 years, I have gone to visit my son's grave on the anniversary of his death and stayed each year with the same friend in Vermont. When my children and I lived in Madison, we were so close to one couple from a town two hours away that they spent the night every Christmas Eve and shared Christmas morning with us. For me, it has always been loving long that mattered, not having 1000 friends on Facebook, none of which are of any consequence.

Only my friends and my children broke through the armor entirely. For me, in my life, my most profound relationships have been with them. Looking at my children as babies, I sometimes recalled the line from Jean Valentine: "You, with no sense of giving/ Brought all the dangers I no longer dared." I have no decent defenses from my children. Once when I was exhausted, my toddler daughter head butted me in the middle of the night, and I swatted her diapered butt. I was immediately filled with remorse. Other than that, I have never struck my children. I have never called them names although once, I must admit, I came close and told my teenage son he was *acting* like an idiot. Profound remorse followed that too. A long, long way from perfection as a parent, I nonetheless can say with certainty that I was not my mother, and that is what I wanted most.

My mother's gifts to me were not always intentional, but there were gifts, nonetheless. She had strength and stamina. No one who ever spent time around my mother thought women were weak. She was who she was, and her capacity for subterfuge was minimal. If my father's kindness and warmth were qualities I wanted to emulate, my mother's narcissism and cruelty were equally educational. It is easy to be your parent. It is not that hard to be the opposite. What is difficult is to be neither. I have never made it to that third transcendent level. My life has too many reactionary qualities to claim I got away from her entirely. Still, the need to be different from my mother has left plenty of good territory to explore. She seldom troubles me now. But the fact that my father let her torment us so, the fact he could have protected us and didn't, that continues to hurt. My father could betray me because I loved him; she couldn't because I didn't.

Chapter 5

The Country Doc

> Self-respect is something our grandparents, whether or not they had it, knew all about. They had instilled in them young, a certain discipline, the sense that one lives by doing things one does not particularly want to do, by putting fears and doubts to one side, by weighing immediate comforts against the possibility of larger, intangible, comforts. It seemed to the 19th century admirable, but not remarkable, that Chinese Gordon put on a clean white suit and held Khartoum against the Mahdi; it did not seem unjust that the way to free land in California involved death and difficulty and dirt.
>
> —Joan Didion in "On Self-Respect" from *Slouching Towards Bethlehem*

The strongest and most repetitive memory of my childhood, over 60 years later, is still the sound of the side door opening and closing multiple times in the night. My father was a country doc who along with a handful of other docs covered all of Carteret County, North Carolina, in the '40s and thereafter until an influx of docs finally came. These early docs worked all day and did house calls most nights. Cell phones were not a neuron firing in the brain of a technician at the time, and people in the poorer parts of the county often had to drive somewhere to access a land line. "Down East" had particularly poor communication. My father would come back from a call Down East, 30 miles of winding road away, and I would hear my mother meet him and say, "You've got to go back," there being no way to reach him on the way or at the previous call to tell him he had another call not far from the first one. Back he would go. This routinely happened multiple times in one night. His heart began to give out in his 40s.

Confronting Malice

When I first wrote this chapter, I found myself with a handful of anecdotes and a feeling I had lost my father somewhere in them. It was not just the things he did, although they were remarkable, but it was something about who he was that shaped me more than any other influence in my life: he was a mensch and his character marked all of his children. My siblings and I have disagreements about my mother, but no one fights about my father. When I was grown, my father and I had been drinking one night and he said to me, "I feel like I have loved you for a thousand years." I thought it was creepy at the time and out of character until one day I looked at my small children and thought, "I feel like I have loved you for a thousand years." He had the capacity for a remarkable kind of unconditional love that my siblings and I could only emulate. Had I turned out to be an axe murderer, it would have broken his heart, but he would never have deserted me. No one in my life has ever loved me like my father did, nor am I the only sibling who would say that. The first morning after his death, my sister heard footsteps on the stairs. My father, who lived across the street, would always come over and check on her children first thing. "What is that?" she said, startled, to her husband. "Oh, just your father checking on the children," he said sleepily without surprise. Nor would any of us say it wasn't so. My mother, on the other hand, told me she would put a cold finger on the back of my neck if I sold any of her rings after she died. I knew my mother well, and I kept the rings.

It was improbable that my father should ever have been a doctor much less the local legend he became. His people and my mother's people were fishermen who did a little clamming, crabbing, and farming for fresh vegetables on the side. They came from Down East, a section of the North Carolina coast which culminated in Cedar Island, which is technically an island but accessible by bridge from the mainland since 1985. Until a decent road was built to the rest of North Carolina, the small villages in the Down East area were as isolated as any in the country. "We were poor," my father said, "but everybody had the same thing, so we didn't know it." Without

Chapter 5. The Country Doc

television or regular communication with the rest of North Carolina, there was nothing to compare themselves to. When I was a child, I remember being told that researchers from the University of North Carolina would go Down East with tape recorders because it was the closest thing to Middle English left in the world. Certainly, the brogue was strong enough to constitute a dialect.

My mother's father was Captain Charlie, a well-known duck decoy maker and fisherman from Stacy, North Carolina. He was born in 1886 and remembered the tall, square-rigged sailing ships that regularly plied their trade up and down the North Carolina coast on their way north and south. He also remembered a stormy night when he was 10 when he was taken down to the sea by some men in the village who put a lantern on a horse's head. The horse, of course, didn't stand still as a statue and so the lantern bobbed up and down with its movements. My grandfather didn't know why they were all standing there until much later. The local men were "land pirates" who misled the tall ships about where the lighthouse was during storms. The ships would wreck and split apart. The next day the men would salvage the goods that drifted up on the beach. Often captains tied themselves to the mast with a money belt around their waists if they had already sold their goods. How many of the townspeople were land pirates? I have no idea, but I suspect from the fact that they took a 10-year-old boy with them that they did not carry out their activities in secret. Some of my folks came from Portsmouth Island, not far from Ocracoke. I have been there and seen a picture of men in rain gear risking their lives pushing a skiff out through driving rain and hurricane-force winds to rescue some poor seamen in trouble. I can't quite fit together the land pirates and the rescue brigade.

My father's father, Papa Mac, was a kind and gentle man who died when I was young. I barely remember him. My father's mother had eclampsia during a pregnancy which brought seizures and left her blind for two weeks. She was never the same after that. It was this event that made the fisherman's son want to be a doctor.

But wanting it and finding a way to do it were not the same. The natural path was to be a fisherman like his father. As a teen, he went clamming with his father, having bought his first clamming fork. My father said it cost $25, and it would take all summer to pay it off. His father raked a large number of clams that day compared to my dad who found the work backbreaking for little gain. On the way back in the skiff, my father sat brooding and finally stood up and threw the clamming fork into the water. Papa Mac jumped up and said, "Son, what have you done?" My father had thrown away the means whereby he could pay off the fork. He had no fork, but he still had the debt. My father told me he thought if he kept that clamming fork he would never "amount to anything" so he closed the door. Of course, there was still the matter of the debt, and he somehow managed to get back and forth the 20 miles to Beaufort that summer to work on the Menhaden boats. Almost everyone, if not everyone else who worked on those boats, was Black, and Black people were not treated well in the South in those days. If my father thought clamming was brutal, the work on the Menhaden boats was worse. The work was hard, and the men got little sleep. There was a point where he came home and slept for 24 hours straight.

Atlantic had a tiny high school at the time but my much older cousin told me it was sending more people to college than any other school its size in the state. Somehow, by hook or crook, my father managed to get into Wake Forest. His older brother, a carpenter, sent him $2.50 every other week. When it was time to graduate, he owed Wake Forest money, and the school had a policy of not forwarding any transcripts unless all monies had been paid. My father made an appointment with the president and told him if he did not send the transcript to the University of South Carolina Medical School where he was applying, he would never be able to pay the debt, but if he did my father would pay the school back and more. The president sent the transcript. My father paid the debt and sent me to school there.

But the letter from University of South Carolina Medical School contained a blow: the school rejected him. In response, my father hitchhiked down to the medical school to ask them why. They told

Chapter 5. The Country Doc

him his score on an entrance test was too low and showed him. My father said the two numbers had been transposed and what they showed him was not his score. It turned out to be true, and my father got into medical school.

Years later, when I first applied to Harvard Graduate School, I too was rejected. I thought it would do no good, but in the tradition of my father, I made an appointment with a professor on the admissions committee for that department and asked why, something that would be impossible today. I don't remember much about the meeting, but they let me in.

A young doctor fresh out of medical school in 1941 knew he was headed to the war. As he waited for his orders, he had a dream. He dreamed he was sent to England, not a surprise, and that he was quartered in an old sailor's home. He went upstairs one day and found a picture of some cancan girls dancing. The dream was so vivid he woke my mother up and asked her to write it down. And yes, my poor scientific, practical, no-nonsense father had to cope with the dream coming true right down to the picture.

While he was in England, he led a five-mile convoy at night when all the road signs had been removed and the houses were dark with blackout curtains to confuse any Germans invading. GPS had not been developed and wouldn't be until 1973. My father led that entire convoy up a blind alley that dark night. As he walked back along the line of trucks backing up, he heard a soldier say, "What idiot did this?" My father didn't defend himself or call out the soldier. Instead, he said from the darkness, "Some damn fool," and kept walking.

He landed at Normandy on the second day of D-Day and said it was the hardest thing he ever did in his life. No doubt that was true, but if so, entering a concentration camp for the first time and finding how the Nazis had treated the prisoners could have been the second hardest. It affected him all his life. Sometimes I would see him looking at a book on the concentration camps with such a puzzled look on his face. He told me when they liberated the camp, the Nazi guards used flame throwers to kill as many prisoners as they could, right before they fled, for no reason at all, he said, "just meanness." He never understood it.

When my father came back from the war, he opened his medical practice in a small town 20 miles from where he first grew up. He had the first integrated waiting room in the county. He told people who didn't like it that they could find another doctor. He didn't take appointments. No matter who you were, you waited your turn. My father never pandered. Am I suggesting that my father, a born and bred Southerner, wasn't racist in the '40s and '50s? Racism was in the water in the South at that time, and I don't think anyone who lived there escaped it entirely, but he had learned respect for the Black soldiers he fought with, and he had less racism than most. He was invited to join the John Birch Society in Kinston, a new organization, founded in 1958, which, for some reason, was popular with doctors in his area. While it focused on anti-communism and the threats of "globalization" elsewhere in the country, its opposition to civil rights was a main attraction in the South. Colleagues invited him to come to meetings, but he said he wouldn't get involved with "that mess" and refused to go. My father never took his colors from his context. He set his own course in a singular way.

My father was a true country doc, as much a psychologist as a medical man. When he couldn't find anything wrong, he would ask his patients what was going on in their lives. One anxious woman reported her in-laws were living with them and it was driving her crazy. The house wasn't that big, she said. My father said she should get a trailer, put it on the property, and move into it with her husband. She did and as her anxiety eased so did her symptoms. He considered this approach an integral part of practicing medicine.

As the years went by, he delivered mothers and their daughters and even their granddaughters. Children he had delivered who had other doctors closer drove back to Beaufort to have him deliver their own babies. He was a gifted diagnostician. He diagnosed a rectal cancer in a friend during a routine physical and referred him to Duke. The technology at Duke found the cancer but the specialist

Chapter 5. The Country Doc

himself couldn't feel it, and he told the man that if he lived, he would owe his life to my father. So did many others.

Have I lost him again in the anecdotes? It is harder to describe his presence and his impact on his children and many others than it is the things he did. He was the kind of father who came through the door and threw his arms wide. His young children would all come running and fly into his arms. I have never felt safer than I did as a four-year-old sitting on my father's lap. His major flaw, as far as his first three children were concerned, was that he loved my mother in the same unconditional way he loved us and wanted us to love her as he did. It turns out you do not have to be good to be loved and this odd couple proved it. He would defend her against all comers. Once out with friends, a woman, no doubt after several drinks, asked my father if he regretted his choice of mate. (My mother was well known in the community.) In reply, he gave a long-winded speech about how my mother was all he ever wanted, and he meant it.

As noted earlier, the research suggests if a child has one person in their life—a parent, a teacher, a mentor, a coach—who loves and supports them, they can grow to be a reasonably healthy adult. The quality of the support is important too. Perhaps it was not just that *someone* loved us, but it was the character of the man who did. Joan Didion wrote in my favorite essay of all time, "On Self-Respect,"

> In brief, people with self-respect exhibit a certain toughness, a kind of moral nerve; they display what was once called *character*, a quality which, although approved in the abstract, sometimes loses ground to other, more instantly negotiable virtues. The measure of its slipping prestige is that one tends to think of it only in connection with homely children and with United States senators who have been defeated, preferably in the primary, for re-election. Nonetheless, character—the willingness to accept responsibility for one's own life—is the source from which self-respect springs.

My father had self-respect. He knew the price of things, and he was willing to pay. He smoked three packs a day from age 10 until age 40, when his heart began to tire. His doc told him he didn't have to worry about lung cancer in 10 years; he would have a heart attack long before that if he didn't quit smoking. He said to me he looked hard at his life. He had young children and a wife who could not support them. He threw the cigarettes away and changed his diet radically. His vegetables were cooked in water from then on rather than the Southern way in oil. They were perfectly tasteless; the smells must have wafted down the table from the dinner the rest of us ate. He had a temper and, somehow, he found a way to circumvent it. One night, at the height of his battle with cigarettes, he asked my mother to go buy him a pack, apparently needing her to collude. She went into the kitchen and filled an iced tea glass with vodka. She came back and said, "Here, drink this." He said he was so angry he drank the whole glass and passed out. It proved to be the continental divide of his battle with cigarettes. It became easier after that, although not by much for a long time. He would sit at his desk and make a decision not to smoke for the next five minutes. That was all he could promise. And then when those five minutes were up, he would make a commitment for another five. He did this for months on end. For years he fumbled with his breast pocket when he talked, looking for the missing cigarettes, but he never smoked again. He lived to see all of us grown.

He could do hard things for many years, literally working day and night, and often accepting a peck of beans or squash as payment. He didn't refuse to go at 3 a.m. because someone owed him money, and he didn't feel sorry for himself for working so hard. He came from stock who pursued their trade on the tumultuous seas of the North Carolina coast in all weather. He lived a life of purpose, and he taught me that a life of purpose was a good life.

I confess that the selfie/social media culture of the youth of today has always left me baffled. Who are these young people who seem incapable of weathering any hardship and don't seem to think they should be asked to? When my father walked the eight and a half miles from Atlantic to Stacy, North Carolina, at night to see my mother before they were married, he walked in the middle of

Chapter 5. The Country Doc

the road to avoid the rattlers, copperheads, and cotton mouth water moccasins that I can personally attest filled the North Carolina marshy coast. Despite a snake phobia all his life, he walked those miles regularly at night without lights. It would be difficult not to have a backbone with a father like that. Of course, I stand up to hostile attorneys; my father stood up to snakes as well.

I see him in my mind's eye, barbequing shrimp in the backyard. He had such joy in barbequing and in taking his children water skiing and in watching the sunset. "Have some shrimp," he would say. I would remind him I didn't like seafood, which on the North Carolina coast was harder for folks to understand than a cocaine addiction would have been. He would look surprised. For 18 years, he could not remember that I didn't like seafood. Only idiots didn't like seafood, and I wasn't an idiot, ergo I must like seafood. "Try one of mine," he would say, convinced if I just tried one of his, the scales would fall from my eyes. I emulated him in many ways, but seafood was a shrimp too far. The message was in the joy he had, in any case.

Not all the old-time fishermen loved the sea—they knew too much about its capacity for rampage—but my father did. He would walk down to the dock in front of our house with me in the evenings to watch the water glitter, streaked with the setting sun. We lived across the road from Taylor Creek, and there was a small island called Carrot Island across Taylor Creek where banker ponies ran wild. "There isn't a prettier place on the planet," he would say. It was one of his many lessons in practicing gratitude, although the term was not current until many years later.

He died in the new hospital, in an intensive care unit that bore his name. I say again, how can you not have a backbone with a father like that? How can you not seek a life of purpose? He didn't just light the spark; he was the spark that lit me.

… Chapter 6 ⇒

How Psychopaths Think

"Just to see him fly."

I have made a point of interviewing and assessing more than my fair share of antisocial men, psychopaths, and sadists. It is not the lost souls who are unlikely to reoffend who have interested me but the professional purveyors of harm. Perhaps my history with my mother and malice lite played a role. The ultimate in malevolence are sexual sadists, but psychopaths too leave an impressive trail of misery behind. Psychopaths commit calculated and dispassionate crimes for personal gain or for dominance that make them recognizable—if you ignore the charming demeanor that some have. But recognizing them and understanding them are two different things. It's harder than you think to make sense of them. They lack a conscience and often enjoy the violence or the scams they perpetrate. They aren't necessarily sadistic—only if it interests them. They aren't necessarily sex offenders or serial killers or even violent—although those who go to prison are four times more likely to commit a violent offense in the first year they are released than any other offender. Basically, they do whatever they want to do without being hampered by conscience or commitment. Many are check forgers and burglars and con men—although some are CEOs and politicians (and con men). Simply put, they aren't one bit sorry for harming others, although they can turn into Meryl Streep crying with remorse when it suits their interests. Their mantra is "Me first, me second, and me third." They are out for themselves, untethered by attachment, empathy, or moral concerns.

My own professional interest began, I think, when I sat across the table from a veterinarian who committed a series of assaults on

Chapter 6. How Psychopaths Think

13-year-old girls. He abducted his 13-year-old daughter who lived with his ex-wife on the day of his ex-wife's hysterectomy—injecting the child with an animal sedative and then ... nobody knows what then. She lived through whatever happened but has no memory of it. He also went into a YMCA, found a 13-year-old girl alone in the locker room and injected her with an animal sedative. She broke away and got out before he could do anything more. How did he know a 13-year-old was alone in the locker room? Does the word stalking come to mind? A third 13-year-old was at home when he knocked on her door "to ask directions" and then took her captive. Someone came, and he broke off the attack. He denied he had any sexual intentions even though he forced her to strip at knifepoint. I told him that he would not have held the home-alone 13-year-old captive and forced her to strip if he wasn't going to do something to her. He replied, "How do you know I was thinking of raping her? How do you know I wasn't thinking about cutting her head off?"

"Were you?" I asked calmly.

"More that than the other," he shrugged. There were missing 13-year-olds in his area and police considered him a prime suspect.

It was then that it happened. I had the sensation that I was talking with an alien. I saw his words as though they were bubbles in a cartoon—blah, blah, blah. I wanted to freeze the moment and reach across and touch the skin on his forehead—as though I could understand through touch what I could not understand through words. It was a visceral sensation that the man across from me was not like me or others that I knew in some way I did not understand. I could not make sense of him.

There have been hundreds of offenders since then sitting across the table. And each and every time, I try to make sense of what I hear. I listen for beliefs, attitudes, motivations, and especially thinking patterns. For the last 10 years I have worked primarily with high-risk sex offenders who have been civilly committed. They are certainly not all psychopaths but to say there are psychopaths in such settings is to say there is sugar in sweet tea. Ten to 20 percent of inmates in North American prisons are psychopaths and typically at least that high a rate in civil commitment programs. Not all psychopaths utilize sexual violence as a way of dealing with the world, but the ones I deal with do.

I don't know how to prevent psychopathy, and science hasn't gone all that far in identifying the precursors in children—although there is likely a genetic component and we know that callous and unemotional children are at higher risk. Nor would it necessarily help to identify it early. We have no answers for the six-year-old who sets his baby sister's crib on fire or for the 12-year-old who cuts the cat's tail off one inch at a time to see when his parents will notice. But as adolescents and adults they can be managed well or badly, and the difference translates into safer or less safe prisons, into inmates who come out of prison more violent or less so.

Talk to violent psychopaths who are before the court, and they didn't do it and had a bad childhood. If neither of those work, they may talk about the traumatic effect their offenses had *on them*: how they have PTSD from what they've done to others. They dissociated, they say. Even now it's too painful to talk about.[1] But talk to violent psychopaths after the trial is over and after appeals have been denied, talk to ones who have been in prison long enough to get bored and who have nothing to lose, and the story changes. It may surprise most people that violent individuals almost always believe their own violence is justified, no matter what they have done or to whom they have done it. Generally, they agree that violence is an acceptable and useful tool for anyone to use.

In fact, the key problem with attempting to treat extremely violent offenders is that not only do they lack remorse but they also positively enjoy the violence. They get a high from it that one offender said "is better than crack, better than cocaine." Another reported:

> You get a feeling like I want to hurt people. It's like something in me. It's a high like sex. If I hurt somebody it's like having sex. After I hurt somebody, I liked to have sex 'cause I feel good....
> I think everybody gets a high out of violence who fights.... Life is

Chapter 6. How Psychopaths Think

based on taking a risk. You taking a risk right now by being in a room with me.

Actually, I'm not, and the best response to that last sentence is no response at all since such offenders also get a high out of intimidating people. He wants to see a flicker of fear in my eyes. (I use flat affect frequently in interviews to ignore statements or questions when people are seeking to get a rise out of me.) For the record, I am in a room with him alone, sure, but because he is in segregation status, he is shackled to a fixed chair. There's a window in the door and two officers standing outside it. And I am out of his reach, anyway. He has no reason to attack me, but he's attacked a lot of people with no reason, so I am careful. I have respect for his capacity for violence and no narcissistic belief that he would treat me differently than others.

The thinking patterns of violent offenders are not intuitive for most of us. They violate normal social patterns and perplex people who are not extremely antisocial or psychopathic. Socialized individuals believe that everyone is capable of caring about other people, that everyone finds violence, at the least, unpleasant, and that everyone has a conscience. Social reciprocity—for example, the idea that if you do something nice for me, I am indebted and I owe you—is automatic for most of us. It is part of an unwritten social contract and has been found in every society in which it has been studied (Cialdini, 2001). Every society, but not every individual. Psychopaths do not think that way. If you do something nice for a psychopath, his first thought is "gotcha." He (or she) starts thinking about how to get more out of you, not about how to pay you back.

I have interviewed and listened carefully to violent psychopaths for a very long time. Unfortunately, much of what I have learned about violent thinking is depressing. When I do workshops on violent cognitions, I end up upsetting the hell out of everybody. Violent thinking is extremely deviant, deeply antisocial, and very difficult to change. We'll start with Ted Bundy, a man whose capacity for conscience we would all agree was flawed. Bundy denied his offenses until journalist Stephen Michaud and investigator Hugh Ainsworth were able to get him to talk about the murders by suggesting that he had at least studied the murders carefully, since he was being accused of committing them, and, therefore, was in a unique position to "speculate" on the real killer's thoughts and emotions (Michaud & Aynesworth, 1989). Under such a thin disguise, Bundy revealed more about his thinking processes than he had ever done before. One of the more remarkable comments he made concerned a rationalization he used for the murders:

> For some reason, it was a necessary way of looking at things. To say that perhaps this person won't be missed. I mean, there are *so* many people. This person will never be missed. It shouldn't be a problem ... [p. 135].
> So, what's one less? ... What's one less person on the face of the planet? What difference will it make a hundred years from now? [p. 188].

With those comments he revealed he had no appreciation of attachment. He could not imagine that anyone's life would be precious to anyone else, much less that complete strangers might make a fuss if someone suddenly disappeared. He couldn't imagine that a human life mattered.

When Bundy was caught and sentenced to die, he suddenly became a staunch opponent of capital punishment—the man had no sense of irony. It seems that an individual life did matter when it was his own. A rather unpleasant part of my make-up would have liked to interview Ted Bundy at the end. In addition to what could be learned, I wanted to say, "So, Ted, about your death. What's one less? What's one less person on the face of the planet? What difference will it make a hundred years from now?"

The mistake would have been mine. That statement assumes reciprocity—that Bundy understood the concept of fairness, that what is fair for one is fair for all. He did not. There is a story of a proverbial exchange between a police officer and a thief:

Chapter 6. How Psychopaths Think

Why did you steal it?
   A. Because I need the money.

What if someone else needed the money, would it be OK to steal from you?
   A. No.

Why not?
   A. Because I need the money.

There is no sense of reciprocity or fairness in this line of thought. It is not "what's good for the goose is good for the gander" but "what is good for me is good for me." The entire concept of law is irrelevant without a belief in reciprocity or fairness.

Witness one offender I interviewed who stole a car in Chicago and drove to Madison, Wisconsin. He saw a man riding a bike in Madison and remembered a cartoon he had seen where someone hit a bike with a car and the biker flew through the air. He decided to try it, just to see how far the man would fly. He circled the block to pick up speed and hit the bike with as much speed as he could generate. The rider did, indeed, fly through the air. Fortunately, he lived, but spent over six months in the hospital. While he was there, the offender wrote the victim letters blaming the victim for the offender's incarceration. He also threatened two judges gratuitously. "Why," I asked, "did you threaten the judges *before* your sentencing?" I have heard felony-stupid before, but even to me this seemed unusually short-sighted.

"They weren't my judges," he said indignantly. In his mind, why would his judge care if he threatened other judges? He hadn't threatened his own judge.

Lack of attachment and lack of reciprocity go together. It is quite obvious in the example above that the offender had no concern for the life of the rider. If you don't care about other people and have no attachment to anyone, why would you be concerned about treating people fairly? There are indeed offenders who have never cared about anyone. They are found mostly among those with horrific backgrounds, but not exclusively.

An offender I interviewed spoke about his history with women:

> I've been in all types of relationships. It was never going to last. Later I started just fucking them, and they have to give me money. I live off myself. I'm a hustler. I don't depend on anybody. I'm a hustler. I like to add, divide and multiply. I don't like to subtract.
>
> *Were there any of them at all that you cared about?*
> A. About 10 I took serious. The last one was the one who stabbed me in my arm....

Somehow, a relationship where someone stabs you in the arm (or anywhere else) does not strike me as a good relationship. Another man I interviewed had isolated and battered his wife for years. When she tried to leave him and take the children, he abducted her and the kids, kept them for several days and then let the children go. He made her kneel and shot her in the back of the head. When I asked him if he had ever loved anyone he said:

> I exposed myself. I did in some sense. I don't mean any disrespect when I say this: women—you demand some kind of connection. You hunger for something more than a mutual friendship. Eventually they wore me down in the sense that I did tell them certain things, but I did this in a way that if they said something to someone else, I would know who said it.

For the rest of us, intimacy is not defined by revealing information that could be used to check and see if the other person told someone. At least I have never found it in Shakespeare's sonnets or even Dear Abby's advice columns.

I made a serious mistake with this man. He had been in administrative confinement (essentially segregation) for many years and done nothing wrong. He was a model inmate. There was a press to release inmates from solitary confinement and who was a better candidate than someone who had no conduct reports in many years? I was asked to evaluate him and wrote a report that said he could be moved to general population, thinking that if he didn't believe he owned a female, he would not be dangerous to one. But I was wrong.

Chapter 6. How Psychopaths Think

His hatred for women was generic, not specific. He stayed in general population for a few months, then one day walked up to a female guard and hit her in the face with his fist. And that's the world I live in: make a mistake and someone gets hurt. Anxiety goes with the territory.

I used to include a question in my interviews with violent offenders about dating but was met with so many blank looks that I had to delete it. "Do you mean dope dates?" some would ask, puzzled. Dope dates refer to situations where females exchange sex for drugs. Particularly among some gang members who were socialized into gangs at an early age, the concept of using women for anything but sex on demand is foreign. Over and over, I have run into individuals who have never had a relationship with a female that went beyond what they could get out of her. "Rent." one offender said. "That's what women are for. I never, never, never pay rent."

Lack of attachment, lack of empathy and lack of a sense of fairness or reciprocity are key components of psychopathy and make it possible for offenders to commit horrific crimes without remorse. The callousness of such offenders is striking. I interviewed one of the national leaders of a white supremacist prison gang two days before writing this. He has been charged with murder twice in the past, told me that the FBI believes he has committed seven, and admits what is obvious: the toll is higher than the FBI thinks. He talks about his going into black communities and abducting and killing individuals he says were drug dealers. I am not at all sure he was very particular in his selections. I asked him if he ever thought about the victims.

> No, ma'am, not once. They were gone…. I never gave them a thought. I have never had any thoughts about anyone I had problems with…. Never did. Never will.

After that, it was foolish to ask him what effect his offenses had on his victims and their families, but I did to document his answer for my report. He responded, "Never thought about it. It wasn't my problem. I got what I wanted."

The depressing part is how *many* examples I have of offenders talking about how much they are indifferent to or positively enjoy violence. One inmate described it this way:

> I believe there are chemicals released when this is going on. I don't know how to describe it or explain it. I just know it feels good.

Depressed yet? No doubt you, the reader, feel worse now than before you started this chapter. Some days I think I should just accept the fact that my mission in life is to spread anxiety and depression as far as possible. In the workshops and trainings that I give, people listen for that last upbeat note, the one that says, "Yes, this is all very difficult but...." In some areas there is—if not redemption—at least some good that can be done. The child who was locked in a basement and starved for five years is no longer there: she is in a good home with a loving foster mom. If she has brain damage from the starvation and social deficits from isolation, the life she has now seems like a dream compared to the life she had before, freezing and starving in a filthy basement while being forced to eat her own feces.

But when it comes to the deeply entrenched thinking patterns of psychopaths and other violent offenders, what can be done with our present tools is a bit iffier. In reviewing the research, I am not persuaded we know how to make them better, certainly not all of them, and there are some data that suggest current treatment programs actually make them more dangerous. I think far too many programs assume such offenders think differently than they do. They underestimate the tenacity and deviance of violent thinking patterns. Nor do we have ways of getting people to give a damn about others who simply don't. Don't look at me for an answer. I'm just digging in the tunnels. I am nowhere near bringing in the light.

The problem is that if you and I saw a child being tortured, we would probably throw up. If we saw a woman being beaten, we would be traumatized. We would not get a high that lasts for days. We would not understand people who do. It is hard to imagine someone getting a high from strangling a child, but I have a video of an offender whose pupils dilate when he describes it, despite the presence of bright lights in the room. It makes a nicer world to ignore his pupils and try to believe he didn't really get a high from that—discounting what he says—and that he can be treated by helping him develop "a good life." But there isn't anything else that gives him the same degree of satisfaction. As he puts it:

> I'd have to say I did get a high from violent behavior. I got a high out of any controlling and dominating situation. Any situation that I was able to control, I got a high out of. I had, like, an adrenaline rush.... I felt powerful, in charge.
>
> Where, in a consenting sexual relationship, sure, orgasm was achieved, ejaculation was achieved then it's over. But the ... the ... the feeling of power and control lasts. It would last a lot longer. It was always there. And it's something I knew I could achieve at any given point any time. All.... I knew what I had to do. All I had to do was control somebody or dominate and that was there....
>
> The high from sadistic acts is different. It's more extreme. It was more extreme. It seemed to me that committing a sadistic act and having sex involved in the sadistic act just heightened everything more, the feelings, the orgasm, the ejaculation, it seemed to heighten it even more.

Another offender describes his experience of beating women not as a loss of control but as a way to control:

> The first time I remember hitting a girl, she had run into an ex-boyfriend. Instead of telling me that, she tried to play it off like she was with a girlfriend. I found out.... I felt like there was an ulterior motive. She was obviously working against me. And I would snap. I would feel bad afterwards, sometimes during it, but I would have to do it.
>
> It was also exciting, which sounds weird. There was one or two women that would understand that the confrontation, the yelling, the hitting, it was arousing as well. That's hard to cope with. It wasn't hard for me to cope with. I understand it. But to find women who understand it, that's a different story.
>
> *Do you understand it?*
> A. It just makes sense. That's the way I've always.... It's always been me. Violence is—I can't explain it. It's right. It makes sense.

It doesn't make sense to the rest of us and no doubt finding a woman who enjoys having her face beaten in as a form of foreplay is difficult. I'm not saying that psychopaths have great lives full of the joy of violence. Sure, they have their moments, but they also tend to have inflated and unstable self-images which they are forever trying to protect. They are hyper-sensitive to criticism and see insult not only in ambiguous situations but also in downright benign interactions. The ordinary prison-bound psychopath—as opposed to the CEO or psychopathic politician—has woefully inadequate tools for dealing with the world. Violence and manipulation only go so far in dealing with a complex society which favors education and technological expertise. Many psychopaths are likely to spend a lot of their lives in the bottom economic brackets and that's just when they are out in the community. I routinely interview psychopaths who have spent most of their lives in a cell.

But they do have some things over the rest of us. They are immune to the one thing in life that devastates everyone else: loss. With no attachment, there is no loss. With no belief that the world is just or fair or meaningful, there is no faith, no belief that everything happens for a reason, no hope that God will protect them. In short, they have no positive illusions to destroy. They cannot be shattered like the rest of us with grief, as I was shattered with the loss of my 17-year-old son to a car accident one horrific night. In this way and this way only, I envy them.

Chapter 7

Working with Psychopaths

Seeing inhumanity in a human is uncomfortable. It makes us want to minimize, to make excuses, to fantasize that there is more to this person than we are seeing. Just below the surface there must be warmth and love and, yes, grief. There's good in everybody, right? Far too many therapists project onto such people of the lie their own internal states and are controlled like puppets by men whose greatest pleasure comes from pulling strings.

The particular man I am interviewing leans back, puts his hands behind his head, and stretches out his legs. "Why do you make educational films?" he asks. I am quietly irritated by the question. I am at the prison interviewing inmates who have seduced multiple staff members into having sex with them and/or bringing in contraband. I have made other training films on sex offenders: on deception, on sadists and psychopaths, and I want to make one on this. After all, it is an issue that faces every prison in the country. In fact, I do not believe there is a prison in the country—or likely the world—that has operated more than two years without having to walk out a staff member for fraternizing with inmates.

The irony is that the inmates with whom staff become involved are not usually the low-risk offenders who are there for selling a few ounces of marijuana. They are the high-risk offenders, the psychopaths, the ones without a conscience, the ones who know how to manipulate people and groom them. It's simple, these offenders tell me. Just build up their ego. One inmate with a history of seducing staff said, "If you can make a person feel good about themselves, most people will respond in kind. They will do things for you that are a little over the line, sometimes way over the line." Another offered, "The main thing is to stroke their ego. They're all cool. 'I wish I could be more like you.'" Earlier today I interviewed a man who killed his grandmother and two boarders who had the bad luck to be home at the time. He has seduced four staff members by official records. He told me he had "done seven." And he probably has.

The inmate in front of me currently has spent the last three hours telling me how he manipulates staff. The first step is to get the staff to talk about something outside the prison. "If they do that," he says, "they'll get personal." My irritation comes from the fact that he is now trying to run his script on me as though he had never told me how he does it.

I look at him. "I like to make educational films," I say. It is the no-information-answer answer, the one that doesn't impart any new data, but one that doesn't ridicule him or pick an unnecessary fight.

"Yes," he says, "but why?"

No respect at all. I feel like saying, "Hello, do you think I'm a potted plant? You just told me how you do this. For Christ's sake, wait a week before you try it on me." I don't say it. I smile and thank him for offering to demonstrate his technique.

I am always polite to psychopaths. Actually, I am polite to all inmates. The only thing I know for sure in this world is that the way we treat people has to do with who we are, not who they are. The people in the pick-up trucks who raced around a Florida prison with signs that read "Burn Bundy Burn" revealed more about their characters than Ted Bundy's. While only social knowledge and common sense can be read from how people treat those above them, the willingness to abuse power can be read by how they treat people below. Look for the line below, not above. Is there any test of character more fundamental? As Dave Barry put it, "The person who is nice to you but rude to the waiter is not a nice person."

But there is one test more fundamental. Look at how people treat *abusive* people they have power over, i.e., those who give their

Chapter 7. Working with Psychopaths

overlords an excuse to treat them badly. There are some people in our prisons who are frighteningly violent and mistreat everyone around them. It is more difficult than you think to be spit on, to have feces thrown at you, to have to clean feces thrown on walls by inmates who are not ill mentally but ill-intentioned instead. It is difficult to deal calmly with an inmate who just put a pencil through another inmate's eye or stabbed a fellow officer in the head.

Still, such inmates frighten me no more than those in power over them when those guards or staff have a reciprocating brutality just behind the eyes, a tide ready to surge whenever there's an excuse. Most staff I have worked with in prisons are both savvy and kind—too kind, sometimes—witness the rate of staff being walked out for fraternization. But there are a few staff whose brutality matches that of the violent inmates. The only difference is that they wait until they have an excuse to exercise it. Violent inmates inevitably give them one.

But even for those who have no moral qualms about brutalizing men and women they have power over, there are other compelling reasons to be courteous to psychopaths. They may lack a conscience, but they have a hair trigger for narcissistic insult. I know of one who chased down and shot a plumber he had called. The plumber saw him on the porch and asked from the steps if he had called a plumber. The man told him to knock on the screen door. The plumber sighed and called out again. "You're standing right there. Did you call a plumber?" The man told him again to knock on the screen door. "Forget it," the plumber said and turned away. This was sufficient insult that the man got his gun, chased the fleeing plumber, and shot him for not knocking on the screen door. True, inmates sitting across from me would pay a huge penalty and gain nothing from attacking me, but I do not need to give them a reason to want to. Even if one decided not to attack me at that moment, he might go back to the unit and take it out on another inmate or guard. Why make him worse?

A polygrapher told me of his master's thesis. Two groups of

inmates, one of which scored high in psychopathy and the other of which did not, were shown two brief film clips. In one a man trying to escape from a prison was shot by guards (life threat). A second film clip showed prisoners lined up against a wall spread-eagled while guards yelled insults and other prisoners walked by (ego threat). Which would upset you more, being shot or called names? If you answered getting shot would be worse, then you are like most of us who believe that "sticks and stones can break my bones but...."

To get around the issue of inmates lying about what upset them most, they were all wired up with measures of physiological arousal: heart rate, skin conductance, and respiration. That way the researchers could directly examine how upset they were and compare it with their verbal responses.

The results lay at the heart of the problem with managing psychopaths. The inmates who did *not* score high in psychopathy aroused more to life threat than ego threat, just as most people would. There is a reason that a standard torture technique around the world is to drag the prisoner out before a fake firing squad in the middle of the night as though they are going to be shot. At the last second, the prisoner is dragged back to his cell. For those not overly sensitized to assaults on dignity, getting killed trumps being called names.

But the inmates high in psychopathy had a different reaction. They flat-lined life threat but elevated to ego threat to the point that the researchers felt they could not send them back to their units until they calmed down. After all, sending a violent psychopath back to his unit in a state of rage is a sure-fire way of having your research cancelled. Of course, flat-lining life threat was no more functional than over-reacting to ego threat, but it explains why psychopaths take chances every day that could get them killed. They seem to get a high from taking risks.

Psychopaths have been called "aggressive narcissists." A better term might be "fragile aggressive narcissists," for they have notoriously unstable self-esteem and seem wired to find insult where it

Chapter 7. Working with Psychopaths

does not exist. This is not to say staff must cater to psychopaths, only agree and never confront—although many do. But psychopaths will turn an inch of leeway into a mile, and staff members who ignore minor transgressions will soon find themselves facing a major one. Still, there are ways that work and ways that don't. Witness a staff meeting about a particularly troubling inmate as an example of a way that doesn't work. The inmate's favorite pastime was to find ways he could hurt himself and either do it or show the guards how he could have done it, e.g., handing over pills he has cheeked and saved up. He has used these incidents to file a lawsuit against corrections, accusing them of not protecting him from himself.

His latest episode involved a nebulizer for his asthma. It came in a small glass container. An inmate with asthma can't be denied access to his medication, and no one thought it a risk anyway. But he smashed the bottle, then claimed he ate the glass. He was taken to the hospital, but nothing was found. Likely he didn't eat the glass, but he could have, and it is another item for the lawsuit. In the past he has found ways to cut himself, then hold down the vein and twirl around, spraying blood all over the cell. He spends more time in an observation cell where he is constantly monitored than in his own cell. Frequently he has to be restrained.

But that's another legal issue. How long legally can you restrain someone? How long can you keep them in segregation? He's never not dangerous to himself. What is particularly frustrating for staff is that this inmate is not mentally ill. He may have a diagnosis of borderline personality disorder, but there are no indications of psychosis, only antisocial personality disorder and psychopathy. Manipulation is his craft, and he makes the staff dance to the same tune day after day. It is difficult for them not to resent it.

A psychologist is talking about his latest interaction with this inmate. He quotes himself as saying, "I don't believe you because you're a liar." I wince.

The inmate had replied, "But I didn't lie to you."

"Yes," the psychologist had said, "but you lied to other staff.'"

Confronting Malice

This is chapter and verse on how *not* to deal with a psychopath. First, if an inmate has developed a relationship with *anybody* such that he doesn't lie to them, that's progress. Second, it is disrespectful to call him a liar, even though he is, and that disrespect will not be lost on this inmate. Third, the psychologist has gotten caught in a power struggle, which is always a mistake. Winning a power struggle is only marginally better than losing one with a psychopath. Both set up a you-against-me dynamic that will only escalate. The art lies in getting your point across without getting into one. So what could you say?

I know what I would say, but I keep my mouth shut. Embarrassing the psychologist in a meeting is not going to change anything. The warden is here. Legal counsel from central office is here. The psychologist is an old-timer and is definitely not going to change his ways; he is known for them. But he could have said, "Mr. Doe, people tell us things not just by what they *say* but also by what they *do*. We have to listen to what people do, because sometimes people say what they want to be true, what they are hoping to be true, but what they *do* tells us what *is* true. If you say you aren't going to hurt yourself, but you do, it's the doing that lets us know where you are." Correctional psychologists routinely manage inmates by sidestepping power struggles.

I learned early. At one point I worked at a community mental health center that covered emergency for an entire county. I also owned a Thoroughbred with legs of such fragility that if the vet had had a spare bedroom, she'd have moved into it. There was even a time the horse ended up in equine intensive care over a benign tumor that bled out. There is a bumper sticker that reads "Go broke; buy a horse." In my case, you could take that literally. On strictly economic terms one could argue a heroin addiction is less costly than a Thoroughbred. But I am of the opinion that "there are Thoroughbreds and then there are a lot of other animals," so I kept working emergency to pay the vet bills.

For an entire year, I was on call every third night covering

Chapter 7. Working with Psychopaths

mental health emergencies for the entire county. There were virtually no hospitals that would take psychiatric patients who could not pay, so it was extremely stressful. In addition, there was a large number of veterans in the area. Many had seen combat, and no small number were destabilized with active PTSD.

"I'm getting those feelings again," a vet said one night. "I think I'm going to tear your office apart." The answer—which unfortunately took me time to learn—is never to issue commands or orders such as "You can't tear my office apart." Actually, he can, and he will. It is also never to cringe and act afraid. If you do, the cringe will make him high with power and he will escalate just to feed the high.

The answer is to sigh and say calmly, "Well, here's the deal. You can tear my office apart, and then the police will come, and you will go to jail. Maybe that's what you want and that's OK. All I know is that I personally am not going to jail tonight. But if you want to, that's up to you. Or you can sit down and tell me what's going on. You decide."

"You decide." It's a mantra when dealing with antisocial, violent, and psychopathic offenders. If you do not give them choices, they will cut off their noses to spite their faces. They will tear your office apart just to show you that they can. You can weight the choices such that one is more attractive than the other, but you cannot get involved in an "I will make you do this [or not do this]" stance.

I am pretty decent at this, but I have seen people who are better. I once had dinner with a Texas capital murder judge who knew the art. At first, I had trouble taking her seriously. Sitting across from me in four-inch spiked heels and a set hairdo was Southern Lady herself. I fled Southern Lady when I left the South. I just didn't want those stupid dolls for Christmas; I wanted a basketball, and I certainly couldn't wear a skirt to school because how could you play tight end during recess in fifth grade wearing a skirt? Southern Lady and I were never on good terms. But here she was back in living color. The judge was telling me the story of an extremely dangerous, multiple homicides offender whose own attorney was afraid to sit next to him and asked the judge to have him shackled in court. In fact, it was the offender who shot the plumber for not knocking on the screen door. A request from the defense to shackle a client is very unusual, because most juries—maybe especially Texas juries—look at someone in shackles and think, "What? He can't even sit there without attacking someone? Guilty." That is hardly helpful to the defense, so it is unheard of for the defense to ask for shackles. She went on, "Of course, I didn't do it."

It was confirmed. Southern Lady was an idiot. "Why not?" I asked.

"I don't shackle people in my courtroom," she said in the sweetest of Southern drawls.

"What happened?" I asked, thinking the point of the story had to be the mayhem that followed.

"Nothing," she said. "I didn't have a speck of trouble out of the man."

"Why not?" I asked, somewhat skeptically.

"I just talked to him," she said.

"What'd you say?" I asked, finally beginning to see this was not Southern Lady.

"I said, 'Sir, how do you pronounce your name?' He said, 'Demouchette.' I said, 'I will pronounce your name correctly, and I will make sure everybody in my courtroom pronounces your name correctly. I will treat you like a man, and I expect you to act like one. Is that clear?' He said, 'Yes ma'am.'"

She went on. "'Do you see that man over there?'" She pointed to the bailiff. "He said, 'Yes, ma'am.' I said, 'If you so much as twitch, that man is going to shoot you. If he kills you, I'm gonna buy him a gold Rolex watch. If he wounds you, I'm gonna fire him. Do we understand each other?' He said, 'Yes, ma'am.'"

I was in awe. I admit, I've never actually threatened to have anyone shot, but still, I knew she had paired the only two things that will contain a psychopath: extreme courtesy and overwhelming force. Neither one alone would have worked.

Chapter 7. Working with Psychopaths

"Where did you learn to do that?" I asked, enthralled.

She drew herself up to her full 5'2" height and said, "On the streets of Dallas. I was a patrolman, and I was small."

She had learned the art of managing very dangerous people without having to hurt them. She may well have been the only person who was ever successful in managing Mr. Demouchette without extreme force. I have told this story in trainings in Texas and on several occasions have been approached afterward by staff who recognized the case and who had had to deal with the offender in jail and in prison. A jailer told me the offender and his brother were in the same jail at one point. "Between them," he said, "they made 35 weapons. We sent them to the police academy so they could use them in training. It was nothing," he went on, "to walk into his cell in the morning and find yourself facing a spear he had made by ripping a pipe off the wall and attaching it to a shank."

Another officer who knew Demouchette when he was on death row told me he had a unique way of postponing his execution: he would kill an inmate or attack a staff member. I very much doubted what he was saying. Why would anyone that violent be put in a position where he had access to other prisoners? There is a large and well-deserved backlash today against the *overuse* of segregation but there is a legitimate use for it—to protect other inmates and staff. There are assaultive inmates, particularly some with life sentences or on death row with nothing to lose who are too dangerous to be around other inmates. Wouldn't Demouchette have been in segregation if he was attacking other inmates?

I looked him up and found the officer was telling the truth. Demouchette had killed another inmate while on death row, stabbing him 16 times in the chest. He beat and raped another inmate, stabbed two other inmates, stabbed two guards, and twice set fire to his cell. I think the inmates who lived with him would have voted for solitary confinement *for themselves* just to get away from him. Demouchette was exactly as dangerous as his defense attorney thought. When he was executed in 1992 the *New York Times* ran an article quoting prison officials as saying he was the "meanest man on death row," a competition with a high bar.

Other staff from death row told me he was so violent in the prison that when they had to move him from his cell, they would show up with a phalanx of officers in riot gear. And yet, a man who managed to kill one person, stab three others including two officers and rape yet another person while on death row in a maximum-security prison, stood and listened calmly to a death sentence being read by a 5'2" woman with a set hairdo and a single bailiff in the courtroom. No wonder I was in awe.

Chapter 8

The Interview

He has long white hair, set against an elongated pale face that wears the expression of an ill-tempered hound dog—if hound dogs are ever so inclined. He has been civilly committed to an indeterminate term as a high-risk sex offender. Were that my fate, I might look a little ill-tempered too.

It is my job to set the stage for the interview, and I do. I sit across from him in a private, neutral room with the door shut. I wouldn't talk to anyone about private matters with the door open. Why would I expect him to? I am, of course, on camera, but there is no sound recording so someone would have to be looking to see if anything goes wrong. There is still some degree of risk in this because this is a secure facility for sex offenders but not a prison, and there are no guards outside the door. Still, he has not been violent within the program, and I go with the odds. It would only do him harm to attack me, plus he has no track record of attacking staff. I dress conservatively: no short skirts, no open-toed shoes, no chest showing, much less breasts, and I dress up. Respect is hard to come by in prisons and secure facilities. Dressing up is one way I can show he is being taken seriously.

I go over the annual review form, and he signs a consent form that I have discussed it with him. No, nothing here is confidential between the two of us. This is a secure facility. Anything he says can go into the report, if relevant. If he doesn't agree with the report, he can hire his own expert. He has a right to a review every year and so on and so on. This is an annual evaluation dictated by law that each and every civilly committed sex offender is entitled to in this state.

I also go over the particular rules with which I operate. This interview is voluntary. In certain situations, the judge may have an issue with that, but it is not my issue. I am a psychologist, and I'm not going to do an interview with someone who says he doesn't want to do it. I will still do the report, whether he interviews or not. I tell him I hope he does interview because, otherwise, I don't have his point of view and can only rely on official records. The very thought of relying only on official records is alarming for most offenders: they want their say. I explain my computer. I tell him truthfully that I can't remember all my questions without it, and it also ensures that I don't misremember his answers. I tell him he can terminate the interview at any time and/or refuse to answer any questions he doesn't want to answer. I offer him breaks and tell him he can add anything he wishes that I forget to ask. In real-world terms, I am drawing a space around us and pointing out the lines.

There are those who think that you cannot confront offenders if you want to establish rapport with them, but I would disagree. It is being fair and respectful that makes interviews possible, not attempts to ingratiate. My manner is telling him I won't demean him. My bluntness about the limitations of confidentiality and my clarity in telling him he doesn't have to answer every question is telling him I'm not going to try to trick him. These things are important to offenders. I am not trying to get them to lower their guard by fake agreement or indiscriminate support.

His official record starts in the '80s when he was caught for sodomizing a nine-year-old boy. He is indignant when I ask him about it. He didn't sodomize him; he "only" had oral sex with him. He is not a pedophile, he says, because he was only sexually attracted to the children of the women he was seeing, and even then, he notes, only when the women have done him wrong. Well, he admits, they don't have to have actually done him wrong. It suffices if they are "going towards" another man, a criteria that seems a bit loose and open to interpretation.

And so, the interview opens. He plays his initial cards. He didn't

Chapter 8. The Interview

do what he thinks is the really bad stuff, and anyway, he isn't totally responsible for it. He had a reason. The women did him wrong. "Your first offense was against a neighbor child," I point out. Even though in my mind that should pretty much end the discussion of whether he only molested the children of women he was dating, I am not surprised when he ignores the point. "Yes, but ..." he says.

It puzzles him, he tells me, that he only molests boys even though there were often girls in the household also. He hedges when I suggest the obvious: he is sexually attracted to the boys and not the girls. No, that couldn't be it. He wants to think it is all situational.

I press quietly, "But do you think the diagnosis of pedophilia is accurate?"

He replies:

> I argue with the part—I'm still wondering why—I don't go out and look for little boys in a grocery store or a mall. I don't look for kids. I don't get involved with any child outside of being involved with a woman in the household....

But he then answers his own question without seeming to realize it:

> I feel more secure doing something with the women's child than picking up a child on the street. I'm scared if I tried to pick up a boy on the street, I'd be killed.

The confrontation here is within him, and that is a far more effective confrontation than one with me. He knows, he truly knows, that he is sexually attracted to boys, and he knows why he mostly molested kids within his home. It is not simply that he is lying to me and to his treatment group; he keeps trying to sell the lies internally.

I listen carefully, trying to filter the truth from the self-serving statements he makes, from "treatment talk" memorized from the several sex offender treatment programs he has been in and from the cognitive distortions that he uses to keep any semblance of a conscience at bay. It is surprising he has veered off already from "treatment talk" to more authentic revelries: usually it is much later in the interview. And he has veered. It is not treatment talk to say he failed to pick up kids off the street because he thought he'd be killed. It is an admission that he was sexually attracted to boys and that he is a pedophile but only offended in situations where he felt secure.

My job today isn't to catch him in admissions. The courts have already decided he is guilty of a series of sex offenses so a "confession" isn't the main point of the interview. My job today is to figure out what his real motivations are so he can be treated and to determine how much progress he has made. Jon Stewart talked about Sarah Palin's "little box of crazy" that she kept on her nightstand. This man has a "little box of sex offender" on his nightstand, and he seems much more interested in keeping the world from seeing it than looking inside himself.

He admits he is not that interested in actually being treated at present. He doesn't think he needs it, but he wants discharge to the community, and that is only possible if the program and the courts are convinced he is no longer high risk to reoffend. He has already been sent to the Transition Release Program once, but he stopped cooperating with treatment once he got there and was eventually sent back to the secure side of the facility. Now he wants to skip the transition program altogether and go straight for discharge. Five minutes into the interview, and I have my doubts about that idea.

I understand why he doesn't want treatment. His providers keep pestering him about the difference in his version of events and the facts. We come to another issue where his account and the victims' accounts differ: anal sex.

> I would never have anal sex with a boy because I know it hurts.

I am actually surprised he is denying sodomy. *Many* of his victims reported anal sex. These were boys in different locations, of different ages, who didn't know each other. The offenses were years apart. I am so surprised at his denial that I blurt out:

Chapter 8. The Interview

But you certainly did have anal sex with boys.
   A. I certainly did not. I admitted I tried to have anal sex. John, I tried to, and I said that, and they said if you tried to, you did it.... Susan, I had suspicions she was going around with this other guy across the street from where she lived, so I initiated having sex with John. Oral sex, first fondling, and I tried to have anal sex with him but as little as he was, and as big as I was, I couldn't do it. I couldn't bring myself to the point of sodomizing John because he was too little, and I was way too big. I couldn't put myself to the point that I would hurt somebody that bad.

But he did hurt him that bad. John described graphically how much pain he was in, and he, like another victim, a five-year-old boy, had anal scarring. There is an additional detail. Both boys, five years apart, with no connection to each other, reported that he made them say the alphabet while he raped them. And no, I have no idea why that arouses him.

The reason for the denial becomes clearer later in the interview:

   If I was really doing that and performing anal sex on that individual party, I would probably want to be dead myself, because it would pop in my head what happened to me, and I couldn't see myself—to this day I can't see myself—putting that much pain on nobody.

And this is what he struggles with: the contradiction between his self-image and what he did. Like most antisocial individuals, he wants to see everything he did as justified. In his own mind, he can justify the other forms of abuse; after all, the women did him wrong, or they were thinking about it, or they had at least looked at another man, but he remembers the pain of being anally raped as a small boy himself. He doesn't want to think he is the kind of person who would put a child through that much pain, that he is no better than the guard who raped him when he was a teenager in a secure facility. After all, how can he center his resentment of the world around this guard if he did the same thing?

The pattern starts to unfold. The mixture of truth, lies and distortions starts to settle into distinct layers, like oil and water. Yes, he says he is definitely attracted to women, but when asked about one girlfriend, he says:

> A. I was in a relationship with her. I went to bed with her one night.

Only once?
> A. Yeah.

Why was that?
> A. It only came up once.... You don't have to have sex with them all the time.

But he had sex with her son almost every night. Why he doesn't realize what he is saying—that he was far more sexually interested in the boy than her—is beyond me, but he doesn't.

So, the interview goes: He makes claims based on what he wants me to believe or what he wants himself to believe but looks at me not as though he is pleading for me to believe him but as though he were daring me not to. He knows the records don't match the claims. His last offense was for molesting a boy repeatedly with a co-defendant. It wasn't *his* fault, he tells me. He was living with a 21-year-old male, and the 21-year-old would bring the victim over. OK, so he watched the other man molest the boy, he adds, and yes, well, he did have oral sex with the boy, but the boy stunk and had some problem where he peed all the time, so it wasn't much fun. By the end of his statement, he has admitted what he denied in the beginning.

"How does he find women with children?" I ask. The 21-year-old roommate is an exception. Most of his offenses occurred after he infiltrated families.

> I've always been with low-income women because the women I have met in the bars, they were low income.

But he finds low-income women who need help in other places as well:

> Like Martha, I met her at the Gospel—she was on ADC. She was getting food. That's what she was doing. She suggested I could find someone to

Chapter 8. The Interview

help her with her car. She turns around and introduces me to her son. I should have backed away 'cause that was a red flag. I know now it was a red flag. At the time it was an open door. I could do what I wanted to do with him.

I conclude this section of the interview by asking how many victims he had:

A. Six.

You passed a polygraph after admitting you had 20 victims.
A. I don't remember saying that.

It has been a long way around, but when I ask him again, "So, is it fair to say at that time you were sexually attracted to boys and not girls?" he finally says, "Yes."

Interviewing offenders requires a slow and patient process. I am juggling the records, the offenders' impression management: how they want to present themselves to the world, the bits and pieces of truth that seep out despite the deluge of "treatment talk," and the motivations and affect behind the distortions and outright falsehoods. The obvious analogy is peeling an onion, but it is more like looking at scrambled eggs and identifying the red pepper, the onion, and, oh yes, that little touch of cayenne. It is all mixed together, and it is held together with callousness, shame, guilt, or indifference. And that is the key point. Not every offender who denies the obvious is a high-risk offender. Low-risk offenders deny too, often from shame, guilt, or even fear that if they admit, loved ones will desert them. The job of an evaluator is not only to sort out the truth from the excuses but also to sort out the real motivations from the distortions and the lies. In the end, I need to get at the motor and the brakes.

It really is ultimately that simple. Have you acted on every sexual impulse you have ever had? If so, you are reading this book from prison or a mental ward. All of us have sexual impulses that we have not acted on. You may think your wife's sister is way too good-looking for your own good or your husband's best friend is hot. You may even think the 16-year-old babysitter is drop-dead gorgeous. It doesn't mean you're going to proposition anybody, much less assault the babysitter when you drive her home that night.

You likely have a normal sexual motor—that is, you are attracted to post-pubescent individuals—but you also have brakes. That little area at the front of the brain notes the sexual attraction but goes "Whoa, I don't think so" in inappropriate circumstances. "I don't think so" because of a variety of braking mechanisms: fear of consequences, moral standards, love of family, fear of losing family, common sense. That little prefrontal area may remind your libido that the 16-year-old looks like an adult but emotionally she's a child. The thinking part of your brain may flash in front of you the likely reaction to your cheating and ask you if you really want to hurt your spouse that much and whether you want to be seeing your kids every other weekend. Even if you think you can get away with it, it may tell you that it's wrong, period. That prefrontal cortex area keeps you married, in good standing with yourself, out of prison, and out of mental hospitals by giving you all the reasons, and listing all the consequences, of inappropriate sexual behavior. "I don't think so" helps you regulate your life and make choices as to whom you will be sexual with, under what circumstances, and when. "I don't think so" is an example of brakes functioning properly.

This is assuming you have a normal arousal pattern to post-pubescent individuals, and most people do. In addition, some people may be sexually attracted to children but are horrified by the attraction and have sufficient brakes never to act on it. We don't know a lot about such folks, but there is no reason to think they don't exist.

Some sex offenders also have a normal arousal pattern, but they have terrible brakes. They are antisocial, and if they want to have sex with the 16-year-old babysitter, they rape her when they give her a ride home. Perhaps they want to have sex with their wife's sister. She isn't interested so they rape her too. If they just propositioned adults indiscriminately, they would be lousy spouses, but I wouldn't be interviewing them. The individuals I interview go beyond bad

Chapter 8. The Interview

manners and infidelity and sexually assault individuals to whom they are attracted or they pick on kids.

Where is the little voice that says "I don't think so" for such offenders? It is singing a different tune. The lyrics go "I can get away with it." Or "Fuck my wife. If she had sex with me when I wanted it, I wouldn't have to get it from her sister." Or "The little bitch is asking for it the way she's dressed" which I have heard said about a child who was four years old.

A normal motor is no guarantee of an offense-free life if the brakes don't work, but some individuals have an even bigger challenge: both a bad motor and bad brakes. If the brakes are faulty and the deviant motor is a sexual attraction to children, voilà, we have child molestation. Some sexual offenses are the product of a deviant motor; all sex offenses are the product of defective brakes.

That bears repeating. The brakes are always a problem in any kind of violent or sexual offending behavior. The motor may or may not be. This man has a problem with his motor. He is truly sexually attracted to pre-pubescent boys. He can reduce that with behavioral interventions, but in the end, he probably can't eliminate it entirely, not without medication, so how is he doing with developing brakes? I turn next to treatment questions.

He tells me he has made more progress with Dr. Devine than anyone. When I ask why, he says:

> When I got around Dr. Devine, I learned I could talk to her. I learned something else. I could talk to a female therapist real easy, but when it comes to male, I don't know why but it gets back in the situation: OK, here's another man taking authority over me. He could hurt me.

It is possible that he is saying this because Dr. Devine is known to give higher scores on progress than other therapists in the program, but I doubt it. What he is saying matches what the interview is telling me about his "treatment responsivity" factors. He does better with a supportive approach in which challenge is done with a gentle tone, embedded in a sea of nonjudgmental calm. Devine could establish rapport with Attila the Hun and probably has. She is very much the master of non-judgmental challenge embedded in support. There are some who have made real progress with her after years of languishing on the wards. Her weakness, unfortunately, is that she can't spot a psychopath, and she has been played by some of the best. This man may have the callousness of a psychopath toward his victims, but he is in no way clever or crafty enough to put forth a consistent false persona, a constructed person that holds together for all that it is false. He says something and then almost immediately contradicts what he just said. This man's real motivations leak through his words like water leaking through wicker.

Apparently, I am not as good as Dr. Devine at this. I must not be coming across as nonjudgmental enough for, suddenly, he flares:

> A. You're sitting there disagreeing with everything I say.

When have I disagreed with you?
> A. You haven't, but in your mind you're thinking.

I do have a problem with two different five-year-olds saying you had anal sex with them, and giving the same details, that you had them say the alphabet.
> A. Yeah, and it was the same police officer.

Are you saying he's lying?
> A. You think police are above reproach but they're not. They embellish. He said, "Now I've got you."

But saying the alphabet is not something it is likely any police officer would make up. It is too specific, too idiosyncratic, and it makes no sense. It isn't the kind of thing a police officer would expect a child to say. Additionally, any student of statement analysis would know that his last answer wasn't an answer at all but a deflection. But I don't go after it. I continue calmly asking questions, and the flare is over quickly. I ask him if he agrees with his therapist's assessment that he lacks empathy for others in his group. Later he will tell me how much progress he has made in developing empathy, but now he impulsively admits what she is saying is true:

Chapter 8. The Interview

> I can't understand why I have to understand their feelings. I have enough problems trying to understand my feelings. They don't understand my feelings.

He does at least eventually admit his primary modus operandi:

> Dysfunctional families is one of the main things 'cause I'll hook on to people like that, especially if I find they have children. 'Cause that will bring me right back down to the same area I was before because in time I will molest that child.

I believe him. In time, he will molest that child. Unfortunately, dysfunctional families of stressed, single women are all too easy to find. He wants me to believe he won't go looking, but he will.

At the heart of every single interview that I have ever done is the unstated question offenders think I'm asking: "How could you?" And at the heart of almost every response has been "I couldn't ..." or "I didn't ..." or "Yes, I did but there were reasons ..." or "Yes, I did, but I'm done with it now." The interviews have an almost predictable flow. More than anything, offenders want to answer the question "Whose fault is it?" and most want to press the point it wasn't theirs.

But that's not the question I'm asking. The main question for me isn't whether their parents were alcoholic and beat them, thereby, in their minds, diminishing their responsibility for their behavior. I want to know whether the motor is defective, not how it got to be that way, and I want to know what's wrong with the brakes. I want to know what the chances are they'll do it again. We're at cross purposes here, so I have to get my information sideways, from left-over tidbits that get dropped when offenders are chomping down on the issues of fault and blame and responsibility. I'm a car mechanic, not a priest.

Chapter 9

On Feeling Safe: Where Does Safety Lie?

Safety is relative, never absolute—not for a biological species in a universe stalked by time. Annie Dillard called it when she wrote, "That it's rough out there and chancy is no surprise. Every live thing is a survivor on some kind of extended emergency bivouac" (Dillard, 1974, page 9). But if safety is a myth, the feeling of safety seems essential to normal functioning. Nobody can really say to their spouse in the morning, "Hope you make it through the day. If not, it's been good." The illusion of safety is there for a reason, as you will find out if you ever lose it. Logic never created that sense of safety. It exists within people who grew up feeling safe and who have never been traumatized. For everyone else, there is unconscious denial of the cognitive realization that people have no tenure here, that accidents and illnesses do not knock first. None of us are safe and all those unscathed by trauma think we are.

Despite logic, that sense of personal safety exists in creatures who have had no challenges they could not cope with. After all, as Milton Erickson wrote, the unconscious doesn't read research. It doesn't read newspapers either. It just goes by the way things have always been. If you had "good enough" parents, and you felt safe growing up, you get to keep that sense of safety until the hurricane winds tear through the front door, the mugger pulls the gun, or the X-rays show lung cancer. "What?" we think then. "Why me?" But the answer is "Why not me?"

I have thought a great deal about safety and what makes people feel safe. I have treated offenders and victims both, and while there

Chapter 9. On Feeling Safe: Where Does Safety Lie?

are a number of issues for offenders—sexual arousal, power, control, excitement, coping, distraction, and revenge, to name a few—there is only one for victims: safety. Eliana Gil, a specialist in treating sexual abuse victims, wrote that she began to get somewhere with victims when she realized everything they did had to do with safety.

And so I have found. The young woman came into my office looking dazed and sat as far from me as possible. Of course, I knew what I would normally do. I would start with who she was and why she was there. I would talk about limits to confidentiality if she was suicidal or homicidal. I would talk about fees and schedules. But I didn't do any of it, not to start with. All that would have to come later. I took one look at her and said, "I want you to think of a safe place. It doesn't have to be a real place. Just a place that makes you feel safe and peaceful. It can be a garden. It can be anything. Tell me about a place where you would feel safe." When she just looked at me, I said, "We'll be talking about difficult things here, things that are hard for you to talk about. I want to be sure you have a safe place you can think about if something upsets you. A place that will help you feel calm."

I didn't say I knew enough about trauma and dissociation to think that she had been traumatized somewhere along the line and that even coming to see someone had her dissociating when she walked into the office. I never suggest trauma to my clients. I suggest safety instead. I suggest ways of self-soothing, of bringing their heart rates down and stopping them from hyperventilating and losing contact with where they are. I want them to be able to take a break and imagine a place without fear if the stories they tell are too hard to hold. I don't want to end up as a fellow therapist did, with a woman curled up in a fetal position under the therapist's desk, in a full-blown flashback believing it was 1976 and she was in the middle of a fraternity rape.

Not everyone can come up with a safe space. Sometimes they blink and search their memories and there is a long pause and then I say softly, "Well, can you think of a place where you felt a little *less* afraid?"

But this young lady had a place. She was a professional softball player. (Yes, there is such a thing.) "I'm catching," she said. "I have the backstop behind me, and I've got my catcher's mask on, and there are a lot of people around, watching the game." I breathe a little easier. For her, visibility makes her safe. Being seen. It makes it less likely the offender was sadistic.

Emotional visibility/invisibility—where does safety lie? For victims of violence it differs, depending on the type of trauma and the type of offender. Many victim therapists believe they can treat victims without understanding offenders, but I do not believe that. I believe that different types of offenders and different types of traumas leave different footprints on the minds and hearts of survivors. The average garden-variety child molester tells himself that the child wants to have sex with him. After all, she didn't run screaming from the room. No, she probably didn't. She or he froze because that is the modal reaction of children to sexual abuse, the response to something they don't understand. Like little rabbits in a field, they freeze. But offenders read it the way they want to read it. "He got an erection," they say. "She didn't tell anyone."

Given this is the number one thinking error of nonsadistic offenders, I often ask audiences why offenders think this way. If there is any one thing that is undeniably true in the field of sexual abuse, it is that there is always a reason for any type of thinking error, and we are looking at the king of thinking errors here. There are a thousand ways sex offenders phrase it, but it always comes down to "They wanted it."

When I ask why offenders think this way, audiences say, "It takes responsibility away from him." Really? Does it? Let's assume he's right—which, of course, he isn't—but for the sake of argument, let's assume the child likes being abused. If you came home and your five-year-old was playing with matches, presumably you would ask your spouse what the heck was going on. What if your spouse said, "Well, she likes it." If your three-year-old was playing in the street, would you care if he enjoyed it? If your spouse let your 12-year-old

Chapter 9. On Feeling Safe: Where Does Safety Lie?

drive the family car or play with a loaded gun, would you shrug and say, "Well, as long as he's having a good time"? When it comes to health and safety, we don't care what our children want. We know they don't understand the consequences of behaviors that can damage them in the long run or even kill them in the short. Saying "she wanted it" may take away responsibility for physical coercion but not for psychological harm.

Of course, the long line of victims seeking help for the after-effects of sexual abuse suggests the basic premise in this line of thought is incorrect in the first place. But that's what thinking errors are for. They bridge the gap between what the offender wants to believe and what the reality is. If the offender doesn't pay attention to the child's reaction, if he projects onto the child his own arousal, he can keep pretending, "S/he wanted it."

"Remember all those great times we used to have," the man said to a stepdaughter home from college, a girl he molested all through her high school years. Still unable to confront him, the young woman stood on one foot and then the other, all the time looking at the floor and screaming in her head, "You son of a bitch. You stole my childhood." He didn't see how much she hated it because he didn't want to.

And why not? Why not see the reality, that this young woman hated him, had been suicidal at times, and had gone into therapy because she felt deceptive for not telling but did not tell so that her mother would not be hurt? It is because the garden-variety offender wants to think he is desirable—even to a child. Almost everyone, including nonsadistic sex offenders, want to look and feel desirable to others. Does this surprise anyone? The cosmetic industry in the United States alone brought in $49 billion in 2022. For the average offender, the fact that having sex with him makes the child want to throw up is not a turn-on. He wants to feel sexy, to believe that the abuse is based on mutual desire.

What this means for such victims is that safety lies in being emotionally visible, because when an offender did not pay attention to how they really felt, he felt free to abuse them. When such a victim comes into my office, I know one thing—that the more I understand about how she or he really feels, the safer they will feel. For such victims, safety lies in emotional visibility. This ties in well with therapy because therapy involves exposure in the face of benevolence. Such victims need for someone to know how they really feel. Someone who can't tolerate the therapist knowing how they feel will have a hard time with therapy.

But what about the victims of sadistic abuse? Sadistic offenders want to know how the victim feels. It is the victim's suffering that is exciting. Such an offender will pay close attention, hoping to detect what hurts or humiliates most so he can increase it. Exposure in the face of malevolence makes victims want to run and hide. Never again will it seem safe to let others know how they think and feel. They might use it to hurt you. For such victims, safety lies in emotional invisibility, in hiding thoughts and feelings. Such a stance will preclude intimacy even though therapy, which involves a special kind of intimacy, may be badly needed to ameliorate pain and restore normal functioning: hence the paradox. Imagine you need water to live, but you're allergic to it. Symptoms may drive such victims into therapy, but that doesn't mean they can tolerate it.

Therapists who treat victims of sadistic abuse sometimes discover week by week that their client is getting worse: she's cutting more or drinking more or is now suicidal and has to be admitted to an inpatient unit. With victims of sadistic abuse, one doesn't establish a therapeutic connection to *do* the work of therapy; establishing a therapeutic connection *is* the work of therapy. The ability to tolerate intimacy without fear or dissociation, the experience of exposure in the face of benevolence—that *is* the therapy.

There is often a clue in what safe space is chosen when I ask them to choose a safe place. For a victim of nonsadistic abuse, the safe place might be a garden or even a ballpark, a public space where others might be around. For a victim of sadistic abuse none of those spaces represent safety. The offender is all-powerful. Nothing as silly

Chapter 9. On Feeling Safe: Where Does Safety Lie?

and as ineffectual as other people being in the vicinity can make them safe. The sadist can inflict intolerable levels of pain and humiliation and they have seen how much he enjoys it. If he can find you, if he knows where to find you, there is no hope. "I am in a boat in the middle of the ocean," one such survivor said. "It is a very small boat in a very large ocean. The water is calm for hundreds of miles around so I can see anyone coming and," she added, "I have a lot of high-powered rifles on board just in case."

Oddly, trends and issues that you are not looking for, that are not currently in the literature, are often hard to spot, despite multiple examples right in front of you. Once you know what to look for, you see them everywhere. "It is the theory which decides what can be observed," Einstein wrote (Einstein, 1934), and I had no theory that allowed me to see the differences in those who sought emotional visibility or invisibility until my second husband opened a door I had not known existed. I lived with a man for 20 years who made it his life's work not to be known. To say that he was secretive is to say there is water in the ocean. A minor example: He insisted I always choose the restaurant for dinner when we went out–every single time for years. When I finally started refusing to make all the decisions about such matters, he would say, "I think you would like to go to...."

I was in my late 20s, fresh off a failed marriage to a very nice man who bored me and I him. My first husband and I had little in common but thought we did, living in North Carolina, because we both disliked living in the South at that time. Once we moved up North it became clear our discomfort in the South was all we had between us. But he was a nice, kind, and decent man. There were no children, we had no money, and the divorce was as easy as moving out.

My second husband, by contrast, seemed beyond interesting. Far brighter than I, he, for example, did all of his Yale undergraduate homework for a one-semester engineering class in a 24-hour period, and he was in a Harvard Ph.D. psychology program when we got together. He could play anything on the guitar or piano by ear, rewire a house, no doubt build one, was a remarkable athlete and a fantastic sailor. Did I mention he was gorgeous? I was dazzled, and dazzled, I missed a few things.

At first the deference and concern for what I wanted were flattering. I felt like I mattered, and people will pay a lot to matter. But I eventually understood he was not in the relationship at all. I gave him a synthesizer for his birthday, and he bought earphones so our son and I could not hear him play. He kept all preferences, thoughts, and emotions from me, including which restaurants he liked, and at the end I came to understand how little I knew him. We lived for a time in a small New England town while I worked at a local college and he finished his thesis. We rented a house in an area bordering a lake where well-to-do people from Boston had summer homes. They came and went, and we never got to know any of them; our friends were other professors at the college. The day we moved out, we stopped for gas, and he went into the station. He came out and informed me with satisfaction that he had "told him!"

"Told who what?" I asked. He had run into one of our part-time neighbors in the store and sarcastically told him how much he appreciated how friendly he and his wife had been to us, how much it meant that they had come over to meet us and had us over to their house so many times. The man was understandably confused. As was I. I don't think I had ever even met this neighbor. He had never come over to our house nor had we gone to his. I had no idea that my husband resented the fact that we had not gotten to know him and his wife or that he blamed them. After all, we had not made any effort to get to know them. The passive-aggressiveness in acting out a part whereby my husband mocked and criticized our neighbor for the fact we didn't know him and his wife stunned me. The neighbor couldn't respond because he didn't understand what this total stranger was talking about and didn't realize what he was doing. My husband could criticize him, and he could not offer any retort. But for me the shock was that he had kept his feelings about the neighbors so inside him that I didn't have a clue.

After moving, we knew another neighbor slightly who lived

Chapter 9. On Feeling Safe: Where Does Safety Lie?

farther down our road. It was a private road, and he and my husband worked together to snowplow it. He never complained to me about the neighbor, and I knew of no disputes, but when this neighbor moved out and a new neighbor moved in, my ex complained so loudly to the new neighbor about the old one that I was dumbfounded. To this day, I can't remember what he had against this neighbor, but he went on and on. He did this every single time he saw the new neighbor. Finally, the new neighbor said he was tired of it, that it was all my ex could talk about and that he didn't want to listen to it anymore. I wouldn't know about that either except that I was standing there for several of these rants.

If the FBI came to my house today and said, "Your ex-husband had a second family and five children in Hoboken, New Jersey, while he was married to you," I would be surprised, more at the Hoboken part than anything—he didn't like Hoboken—but not astounded. If they said, "Your ex-husband was a member of the New York City ballet when he was married to you," I would think, "Interesting. I wonder how he pulled that off. Well, he had the body for it." If they said he was an alien beamed down from Mars, I would be downright amazed that there were colonies on Mars.

I do not know all the details as to why my husband was as he was, but I knew enough to know his upper middle-class family was peculiar and enough to know his mother was at least emotionally sadistic to his sister. I suspect his mother was to him as well, and he just learned to protect himself better, becoming at least superficially well-functioning. His sister did not.

If I make it sound like he was a cold fish, he was. I remember thinking, "I am married to someone as gorgeous as Michelangelo's David and about as warm as the marble." But if I make you think I was a good marital partner, I wasn't. I didn't handle the situation well. I became needy, asked him to do things for me continually because it was the only time we spent together. I yelled and nagged and muttered to myself continuously "I thought marriage would be more than this" for years on end. I became a workaholic, wrote books, and did workshops throughout the country, which was horrible for our son because my second husband was a workaholic too. I tried to fill the void my marriage had opened up in me and was counting the days until our son went to college so I felt I could leave my husband without upsetting my son's world with a divorce. I counted days for eight years.

I lived with a man whose sense of safety lay in emotional invisibility and never saw it for 20 years. I even had fair warning from, of all people, an astrologer whom we went to see when we were still dating. We were young and mildly interested in New Age culture and thought it would be fun. It wasn't. The astrologer told us not to get married. She said my husband would project his mother and sister onto me and respond to me as though I were them. She didn't seem to like me very much either, and while I can't remember the words, I remember thinking she saw me as demanding. But while it did my failed marriage no good, the experience of living with an invisible man opened up a line of thought in me. I began to see that not every victim I was working with felt safe with the being-known qualities of therapy. Some folks' only sense of safety lay in hiding from others. I began to see the paradox this created for therapists as well as for friends and family.

If you know such a survivor, edge closer softly. Take your time. Speak of the easy and familiar. No New Age instant intimacy. Let them reveal what they want to reveal when they want to reveal it. No showing off with interpretations or insights they haven't thought of first. Don't pounce on things that seem obvious to you unless they are obvious to them. They will panic if you seem to know more about them than they have consciously chosen to reveal. Mostly, just stand still and quietly wait. Wait for them to look up, to sit a little closer, to talk of things that hurt and then just sit still long enough for them to know you aren't going to betray or hurt them or use that knowledge against them. And if you betray that trust, may the gods that be have mercy on your soul.

≡ CHAPTER 10 ≡

Grief for a Lost Son

Why talk about personal loss and crippling grief in a memoir of a professional life? Because first of all, there is no better contrast between psychopaths and the rest of us. Loss, and our reaction to it, draws the boundaries between psychopaths and the rest of us with the sharpness of a scalpel. It is true also that those of us lucky enough to have meaningful jobs—and they are rarer and rarer today—know that our personal lives inform our work, make it possible to do some kinds of work and unable to do others. I grew up equipped to deal with the hostility encountered in court and the malevolence encountered in offenders. But for a long time, I also had the capacity to work with small, suffering children. And then I lost it.

I lived and worked in New England for 20 years, all through my second marriage and the birth and rearing of my first son. I worked with victims and offenders although I saw more victims. There simply were more victims: each offender tends to make more than one, and some make astronomical numbers. Because I had a master's degree in child study in addition to my Ph.D. in clinical psychology, I often evaluated and treated very young victims, and I went to court on cases with preschoolers. If you want a hard job, apply. Prosecutors generally win most of their cases overall, but the younger the child, the less likely it is for juries to believe them. Send a man to prison on the word of a four-year-old? Juries waiver, and at least one or two will hold out. Because of this most prosecutors are reluctant to go to court on the word of a preschooler. Even if they believe the child, they rarely think that a jury will.

But the problem with very young child witnesses is more than a jury's blank faith in the adult's word over the child's: the problem is that young children don't have abstract reasoning and they don't understand court. They really don't know why they are there, and few children will hold forth in a large room filled with strangers. Very young children talk about things when they feel like it, not in response to a question. The three-year-old may climb out of the tub and horrify his mother by saying, "Will you suck my penis like daddy does?" But dress them up, take them by the hand and walk them through the door to a gigantic room with everyone staring at them and—good luck. As for children under four, it's open season. Unless there is a witness—and who molests kids with a witness?—there is nothing the courts can do. Very few cases leave medical evidence. What evidence does fondling a child's genitals or forcing them to perform oral sex leave behind?

The day came when I couldn't do it anymore. I couldn't do it because I couldn't cope with the pain in those small faces. I couldn't treat children who were forced to spend weekends with a parent whom they said over and over was hurting them. I couldn't see the pictures they drew of anal sex. I couldn't do it because a sadist won his court case and custody of his four-year-old back, and I had never seen a more frightened child. But most of all, I couldn't do it because I had changed. Because I had been eviscerated by the death of my son in a car accident, and I no longer had that much to give.

I lived in New Hampshire at the time, but I was in Boston for a workshop when my world imploded into a confused ball of pain and disbelief. I was back in Brookline, a suburb where I had lived while going to graduate school, for a workshop on hypnotism. My bookshelves in New Hampshire were filled with the works of Milton Erickson, and I was entranced with the possibilities of using hypnosis to ease pain of all sorts, mental and physical. I wanted to add it to the techniques I used as a psychotherapist.

The day itself broke Boston sunny, and I went for a morning walk. I lack the inherent sense of spatial relations that many have. If I have the genetic capacity at all it has not been "expressed," as they

Chapter 10. Grief for a Lost Son

say. Had I been born an Aboriginal person at a time when spatial skills were essential for finding water, I would not have lived past my first foray into the desert. In short, I knew I was in a bed and breakfast in Brookline that I had found online but had no idea where I was in relation to any landmark I knew when I lived there.

As I walked through streets, I stopped short at one corner. There was a street I did remember from long ago—17 years, in fact—back when my second husband and I had our one and only child together, a boy. We had lived with other students in a house in Brookline then, and if I wasn't mistaken, it was on this street. I headed up the street and stopped in front of the familiar house on a sloped site. Suddenly, I remembered vividly bringing the newborn home from the hospital to this house. I even remembered the clothes I had worn, an orange-and-black-striped wrap-around skirt that tied, the only non-maternity clothes I had big enough for a new momma bulge. I was filled with unfettered joy standing there in the sunlight looking at the house as I remembered carrying the baby up the sloped pathway to the front door. I had no idea that at that moment death was crawling closer and closer, stoplight to stoplight slowly in the Boston dawn.

I had had plenty of premonitions of disaster in the couple of years before this. I had been filled with an escalating anxiety that time was running out, but no idea what time was running out for. But that day when the personal apocalypse finally hit, I was clueless. I slept through the night, woke to find the house where it all began, and felt nothing but joy at the memories of his birth. Was it coincidence that I found the house I brought the newborn to on the day he died? Was there some alpha and omega meaning that my subconscious put together? I never knew what to make of the fact I was staring at his first home, filled with joy and remembering his birth, while my husband was driving toward me to tell me our son was dead.

I walked back in the sunshine, my brain running through memories of my son as a baby and a toddler. I was so preoccupied I barely noticed when I got back that the proprietor of the bed and breakfast was nervous, her manner very different from when I left. To the extent that it even registered, it never occurred to me that her nervousness might have anything to do with me or that she might have received a phone call while I was out, asking her to keep me there if I tried to leave before my husband arrived. I went up to my room and climbed in an easy chair to read while waiting for breakfast.

The door to my room opened. It was my husband. He was supposed to be at our home in New Hampshire two and a half hours away. We were not doing well as a couple. Our marriage had diminished over the 20 years until it was little more than the carcass of a marriage. Still, we were trying, and I smiled when I saw him. My first thought was what a nice surprise that he had come to see me. Then I saw the look on his face and time stopped. He crossed the room and fell on his knees in front of me, holding onto my thighs. "It's bad," he said. I knew immediately that he meant our son, but for a second, I had hope. "Bad" is not necessarily irredeemable. "Bad" might mean a lengthy hospitalization. "Bad" could be a lot of broken bones. "Bad" might be a recoverable coma. But then my husband said, "Corey's dead." He didn't tell me then that Corey had dropped his girlfriend off after spending the evening with her and my husband at the house. He didn't mention the winding back road at night where he hit a tree and died. If he said anything after that at all, I don't remember. The words themselves created such a seismic shock I immediately hallucinated them. I saw them written in script in the air in front of me. I pushed my husband away. "Go away, Greg," I said. "I'm having a really bad dream, and I need you to leave now so I can wake up." He just held on harder and started crying.

After that I don't remember anything until I was downstairs. I had packed, I think, or tried to. Maybe my husband packed. I do remember that my addled brain was trying to cling to some semblance of normalcy, and I became fixated on the idea that I had to tell the workshop leader I wasn't coming. I couldn't remember his name or how to reach him, however, although I knew him and his number was in the papers I had with me. Finally, I remembered his name

Chapter 10. Grief for a Lost Son

was Brown, and I tried to look him up in the phonebook. I opened the phonebook but couldn't remember where B was in the alphabet. It seemed so complicated to find B. Nor could I read the words in the phonebook. They were in some undecipherable code. I kept turning the pages looking for B until the proprietor gently took the phonebook out of my hands. Next, I remember having trouble breathing and thinking how hard it was to get from one second to the next. How would I ever get through years and years of all those seconds?

We drove home. We had two cars there and both drove separately, a dangerous and irrational plan. Neither of us was sane enough to think of any other way to do it. I don't remember getting out of Boston. I do remember one or the other of us stopping every few miles because we couldn't drive anymore. One of us would signal the other and we would stop, get out of the cars, and cling to each other sobbing. The first thing we did on getting back was drive straight to the garage where his car had been towed—another mistake. He had hit a tree and his car had caught on fire. The sight of the burned-out car was another trauma.

We never knew why he hit that tree. He was coming back from taking a date home. They had been at the house, and my husband said that they were having fun throwing strawberries at each other. He had a good day. He had just gotten into the Berklee College of Music. He was gifted in music, like his father, and he was so excited about Berklee. But he had also gotten into drugs and was just starting treatment. Did he kill himself? He had no drugs in his body, the autopsy said. Was it simply inattention? Did he reach for a cassette tape and miss the curve with the tree next to it? Was he singing or working out a new composition in his head? The mystery of why he hit that tree is like a parasite in my brain that I cannot ever kill. It means there can never be any closure, and I will always be left wondering.

This was late June, and after that, there are only flashbulb memories of the rest of that summer. I saw isolated pictures in my head of the service, the gathering on the lawn afterward with no memory of what transpired before or after. I remember friends and colleagues filling the house. I have one memory of colleagues from the department sitting in a circle in the living room while I just put my head on a friend's shoulder and wept. Everyone looked on uncomfortably, wondering if they were helping or hindering by being there. I remember going to pick out the gravesite, starting to faint when I got out of the car and having to sit down on the hillside next to it. I have one flashbulb memory of a part of Corey's service and another of talking to a friend outside afterward. I remember later in the summer walking by a restaurant with a glass wall and feeling like the diners were in another dimension. They talked and laughed, and it seemed they were in a different world. I saw an image of myself floating like a balloon above the earth with one frail tether connecting me to it. I remember going to that same restaurant to meet a friend later in the summer and tears running down my checks as we talked. I don't remember even noticing how the other diners reacted. I wouldn't have cared if I had. I didn't do anything but cry that summer, no matter where I was. The rest of the summer is gone. It just didn't seem to encode. All I have left of those memories are the mental snapshots.

Before my son died, had you asked me what grief over the loss of a child was like, I would have said terrible suffering was involved. What I didn't know, and had never read, was that the suffering was not just emotional. My brain was addled, in shock, and unable to function normally. The memory loss was only part of it. I had trouble finding words and was almost completely aphasic at times. I couldn't always put a sentence together. My voice was so small I couldn't make it loud enough to trigger an answering machine when I tried to call friends. I had a constant metallic taste in my mouth, which I was told later is a symptom of liver malfunction. I couldn't eat and didn't eat at all for the first five days.

The shock affected my sense of self. I didn't feel like I was a person anymore. I had read of Holocaust survivors saying that, but I had never known what it meant. How could you not feel like a person? You could be devastated. You could feel lost. But you were still

Chapter 10. Grief for a Lost Son

a person. What did that mean? I still don't know what it means, but I know how it feels. I didn't feel like I had a personality anymore or that I was a cohesive entity. To the extent that I had any self-image, I saw in my mind's eye a ragged creature whose entire left side of her body was crippled, damaged beyond repair.

I awoke every morning and there was a single second when I knew something dreadful had happened but didn't know what. That terrible moment was the best moment of the day. After that, reality came crashing in like a tsunami, and the day turned into seconds to get through. My chest felt hollow and fragile. I would close my eyes and imagine wrapping bandages around it to keep it from falling part. With that image of bandages wrapped around it, I would get up and try to get through another day.

The day consisted of seeing friends and trying to talk or sitting outside in the garden and saying nothing. My husband and I went down to see my parents who lived on the coast of North Carolina. We put chairs outside and just sat there looking at the water for most of the day. Eventually, months later, I went back to work. I had to. I thought if I stayed home any longer and thought of nothing else, I would go insane. I needed something to distract me. My husband was caught in his own grief, and neither one of us had enough emotional resources to help the other.

Surprisingly, I was able to focus on other people's pain, to push my lost child aside for the workday. But I was simply damming up affect that flooded the moment I quit working and headed home. My son's death would sweep over me on the ride back as though fresh from a day's hibernation. These were grief attacks, and they would not abate for many years.

There is a reason there are different words for grief and depression. They may be kin, but they are not twins. Depression is a kind of inertia, a feeling of emptiness and despair that can suck all the energy and life out of a person. But grief attacks, and it is like wrestling with an 800-pound gorilla. The grief attacks came reliably on the way home from work, but they also came unpredictably at other times. I would be stable, functioning reasonably well, when I would suddenly feel my mood sliding downhill like an elevator without brakes and then the grief would hit. It was an active attack, an ambush, not a passive sense of depression.

Six months later at Christmas I was suicidal, even more suicidal than I had been in the first few months. My husband had chosen to go on some sort of work trip for weeks around that time, and he had rejoined the theater group his former (maybe former) lover was also a part of. I sat in the kitchen one day debating whether to go in the garage, close the door, and hook the vacuum cleaner tube to the exhaust. I had measured the exhaust. I knew with a little duct tape the tube would fit. I sat there rocking by the wood stove. The duct tape was sitting on the table in front of me. I kept rocking. Going to the garage would have been as easy as crossing a pencil line on the floor. The lack of connection to the world made it easy. My son was gone. My marriage was over. It would likely have ended anyway, but it was certainly not strong enough to survive this. Friends tried but could not understand. Some concentrated on my husband, feeling I was the "strong" one who didn't need their help as much. A few friends stayed away entirely. They had no ability to tolerate being around someone so crazy with grief. I had but one connection. I had finally found a therapist who could genuinely provide a space where I could grieve. I kept rocking. I knew it was a toss-up whether I lived or died, but I didn't care. I only had a vague and distant interest in the outcome. I might go to the garage. I might not. I kept rocking. I kept thinking that God must be a sadist to inflict or allow such suffering. Had I really been sure there was nothing but darkness and the end of pain in death, I would have gone. But facing a sadistic God? I realized after a while I wasn't going to the garage that day. It turned out that day was the closest I came. The one connection with my therapist pulled me to life and the fear of a sadistic God closed the door to death.

After that, even decades later, I could no longer work with abused children. It takes strength and stability to tolerate the suffering that

Chapter 10. Grief for a Lost Son

abused children go through, to listen to the stories, to see the sad faces. It takes emotional control of a type I no longer had. I was triggered by their suffering, and when I was, my affect dropped through the floor. It felt like that elevator again, the one that had lost its brakes. I didn't know that you could feel OK one second and the next be suicidal, but that's what it felt like. I had to do the work I could do, the work that did not overwhelm me and trigger the PTSD that I was trying so hard to keep at bay.

I could go to court and testify about child development or the research on delayed disclosure of sexual abuse. I could counter an expert who testified that beating eight-week-olds with sticks for not paying attention in church was not abuse.[1] But I could not bear the pain in the faces of abused and neglected children. Evaluation and treatment of abused children were out.

Rumi wrote, "The wound is the place where the Light enters you," but I can't claim anything as grand. For me, the wound was the place where the darkness entered that nearly killed me. If I close my eyes and form an image of myself, I still see one whole side of my body as shriveled and damaged, and it's true, I am. But you work around what you can't work through. I never said I was healthy. I never even said I was normal. I am, as Annie Dillard wrote, "a frayed and nibbled survivor in a fallen world, and I am getting along."

The careful reader will note that this chapter does not have the same rhythm and cadence that other chapters have. That is because I am writing *about* my life in the other chapters, and I am *reliving* it in this one. One early reader suggested I rewrite this chapter so that it fit with the others, and I tried, but I was incapable of it. It always came out this way. And why not? After all, it has only been 32 years.

Chapter 11

Three Years Later

I stared at the stucco building debating whether to go in. The sign for the fortune teller, "The Blue Lady," stood side by side with a sign for an accountant. Apparently, they were officemates, albeit curious ones. Not to mention I thought fortune telling was a scam. Well, I thought, I'll go in to see her techniques. She'll say something like "You have trouble with relationships," which could apply to every single human being on earth.

A hunger for the other children I had always wanted had hit me like a hurricane after my son's death, and ultimately it brought me here to San Antonio. My marriage had dissolved by this point. The divorce seemed of little consequence, the marriage had died so many years ago.

If I could not work with small, suffering children anymore, it did not stop the hunger for healthy ones. A fertility clinic I had found there in San Antonio was the one place in the country I could find that would take a 45-year-old woman who was also single. Other clinics would have taken a single woman or an older woman but not both. I was there a day early, because I never trusted planes to get me anywhere the same day I left, and once the donor sperm–donor egg embryos were thawed there was no going back. It was my third trip—the other embryos had not taken—and if this didn't work, there would only be one more trip as the next would exhaust the remaining eggs. On previous visits I had seen the Alamo and the River Walk, and this time with a day to kill, I had headed for the old city just to wander where I had come across the stucco building with the fortune teller and the accountant.

I walked in and sat in the joint waiting room. The accountant had his door open, and I said to him, "Is she for real?"

Chapter 11. Three Years Later

"I don't know," he said. "All I know is that people come from all over the world to see her." I raised my eyebrows at that, at least internally, but thought maybe he was just trying to support her.

Her previous client left, and I went into her office to see a rather ordinary looking middle-aged woman in street clothes. Had I expected a turban and a crystal ball? Maybe. As I sat down, she said, "Who's Rosalie?"

Startled, I said weakly, "My mother?" She looked at me. "You're a counselor. You treat people." More staring. "You write. You've been published." By this point I was thinking about what the probabilities were of randomly saying three things in a row that specific and getting all three right and my head was spinning. I had told her nothing about myself. I hadn't even had a chance to, and I had gone in on an impulse. She had no way—well, no ordinary way—of knowing I was coming. I told her then why I was in San Antonio and that I was both trying to get pregnant and trying to adopt, happy to settle for whichever happened first, if either did. "You're not going to adopt," she said confidently and then took my hand and told me to make a fist. She looked at the side of it. "Funny," she said, "I see multiple births. Do twins run in your family?"

A little over eight months later, I looked over my massive, twin-carrying abdomen at a spoon on the floor, debating whether to expend my energy for the day by picking it up. Stooping over and raising that belly back up would exhaust me. "Well," I thought, "the lady who cleans is coming in a few days. She can pick it up." It would have to wait. I walked by the hospital bed I had rented so I could sleep sitting up as I headed for the car. If I laid down flat the twins were so heavy on my chest I couldn't breathe. My 130-pound frame was now 195 pounds, but I was still working although I had stopped working with children because children required getting down to and up from the floor, and that was not going to happen without the intervention of a crane. I still saw older children who talked rather than played on the floor.

I was wearing the loosest maternity blouse that I had, but

maternity clothes were no longer big enough and I had already popped a button. When I went down an aisle in a supermarket, people sometimes turned around and headed another way. I am at a loss for metaphors to describe the shape I was in: beached whale, Goodyear Blimp, perhaps pregnant hippo comes closest. I was also nauseous and had been for the entire eight months; twins produce more hormones than a single child. I lived alone in the woods at that time, and I would drive to town and sit for 20 minutes in the parking lot of the supermarket waiting for the nausea to subside so I could go inside. At times I never made it inside. At other times, I left full grocery carts in the store and drove home. People who knew all this thought I was having a hard time. I wasn't. Carrying two healthy babies after the nuclear explosion of losing a child just felt physically rugged. I could do physically rugged. Losing a child was like having a lit match put to your eye.

I lost my father while I was pregnant, and I was so tired on the way back from his funeral in North Carolina that I put my head down on the airline ticket counter. The agent looked at me for a moment, then handed me a pass to the airline's club lounge. A federal judge was not so kind. I started bleeding during the trip back and ended up in the emergency room, missing a deposition. The judge fined me for missing it, despite a note from the emergency room doctor, although to be fair he dropped the fine once the case ended.

This particular Friday I was seeing my doctor, and when I did, he informed me that three weeks short of my delivery date, my blood pressure was giving up the ghost. They would induce me on Monday. It was pretty clear the babies were big enough, he added, eyeing the belly that was now so big I had trouble reaching the steering wheel.

So that weekend, I called a friend who was an artist, and she came over and made a plaster cast of my belly and breasts and painted it with swirls of color. I kept that cast for years and wish I hadn't eventually thrown it out. I also informed the caterer I would be going in on Monday. I had engaged a caterer to set up food for the labor. I had had a joint appointment in the hospital in two different

Chapter 11. Three Years Later

departments and had friends there. I knew doctors and nurses would be stopping by to see me, so I set up food for them and a table to hang out. For me this was a celebration. Twenty-four hours after labor began, I was feeling a little less celebratory and had decided I'd forego the natural childbirth I planned in favor of an epidural. When the anesthesiologist did not arrive promptly, I asked the nurse, "Where is he?"

"He's on the phone," she said. "WELL, GET HIM OFF THE PHONE," I yelled. Childbirth is the enemy of polite and gracious exchange, and there are no Southern Ladies in delivery rooms. Later I counted 26 people in the delivery room. My age at 46 alone made me a high-risk pregnancy, on top of there being twins. There were two full neonatal care teams there, one for each baby, a delivery team, and a few friends of mine as well. Finally, one child was born at 4 a.m., but the second—possibly swimming around happily in all that now-empty space—resisted meeting the world until 10 a.m. They weighed seven pounds, 10 ounces, and seven pounds, 11 ounces, each larger than the average single baby. A pediatrician friend said to me, "18 to 22 months, Anna, gonna be a little busy." He should have said, "Birth 'til the cows come home, Anna. Gonna be a little busy."

Literature talks of the tiredness of combat soldiers in war, but few books describe what life is like for single mothers. Of course, I had more advantages than most. I was able to hire help, at least during the day. Many single moms work two jobs to support their child, take whatever childcare they can get—however inadequate—and never see their young children awake as babies. I could and did hire a nanny, a Finnish nurse, and she took care of them all day but, of course, she slept at night. I worked all day and took care of them all night. Despite their size, they were adamant about being fed every two hours and so I was up every two hours every night that first year. The only night my nanny took care of them was once when I was hauled off to the hospital with food poisoning. The night I came home I was up with them.

The kind owners of the office building where I worked offered me a second room for the babies down the hall from the first for $1 a day. I installed the babies and Minna, the nurse, there while I worked, and I rushed down to see them and feed the babies between clients. On weekends I took care of them day and night. I developed the insane idea that I wanted to write a second book at that time. It had nothing to do with ambition. When books are ready to be birthed, they beat in your chest like wild birds until you let them out. And too, writing anchored me. In the confusion and exhaustion of this new life, the one thing that brought me calm was the minutes I could write. Of course, I was tired beyond comprehension, and I was seeing double every night. In the type of logic that only the severely mentally ill and the crazy exhausted know, I decided seeing double was not a reason to stop writing because I always saw double at night, but when I couldn't decide which screen to type on, I had lost it and needed to stop. I was quite pleased with my differential at the time and did not see the insanity it represented.

When the babies were a few weeks old and lying on my bed, I turned around and saw that my daughter looked as though a line had been drawn down the center of her face. One side was puffy and red, and the other side was perfectly normal. The line was as distinct as though someone had drawn it with a ruler. I grabbed the phone and called the emergency room. "Oh yes," they said, "that's Harlequin syndrome. A lot of premature births have it. It's harmless." The babies weren't premature, but my daughter had it that one time. By the time I got off the phone, the line was no longer distinct, and the blotching was fading. But I, who had thought I was coping pretty well, could not get my heart rate below 125 for the next three days.

But if I was physically stumbling around and if there was always fear of something happening to the babies, my head and my heart were nonetheless getting better. I had a life. I had love as well as work. If the old soaring joy was gone, there was still joy. And there was hope. I hoped the kids would be happy. I hoped they liked their preschool. I hoped their five-year-old soccer team won a game. I hoped they found people who loved them like my father loved my mother.

Chapter 11. Three Years Later

But I never hoped the bear-like attacks of grief would go away. What point was there in asking hurricanes not to exist? Half my heart was a shriveled-up mass of dead muscle; half was filled with the laughter of infants. Managing both sides and dealing with people during the day who molested children made me tired long past their infancies. Throughout their childhoods, the most difficult clients I had were men who molested children the same age as my own. That took emotional control, but I had people in my lineage who survived the North Carolina coastal storms and hurricanes—not to mention the Portsmouth Island mosquitoes—and I persevered. I persevered because I believed to the tip of every hair on my head that I was helping to prevent child abuse and that seemed like a worthwhile, if challenging, way to spend a life.

The old life and the death of my son would never entirely leave me, and the best accommodation I could make was a type of PTSD numbness. After I got over the nuclear shock of his death, after the first 10 years when I could take a breath, I settled into a numbed zone of affect where I never went too low or too high. But at least with the babies I had connection.

Chapter 12

On Connection

When my second husband and I were graduate students, we had a 25-foot sailboat that had no radio, no radar, and no motor. Sometimes on the way from Mattapoisett Harbor to Nantucket, the fog would set in. Of course, that area is heavily trafficked with ferries, very large ferries, ferries a lot larger than a 25-foot sailboat. Not having radar meant my husband and I were dependent on limited vision and on hearing to avoid the ferries—not to mention on having enough wind to maneuver—and the hope a ferry's radar would pick us up. It didn't always. Once in the middle of Woods Hole at night, a ferry got very close before its foghorn sounded a loud squawk and its giant eye pinned us.[1]

If the fog was thick enough, there were times even in the middle of the day when we could hear the ferry's fog horns getting louder and louder as the ferry drew near, but we could see absolutely nothing. While my husband steered, I would literally lie on the bow of the boat as far forward as I could get without falling off, straining to see an emerging behemoth. We couldn't tell if the sound of the ferry's motors was rising or if it was dead ahead and would loom over us at any minute, too late to avoid impact, or if it was slipping quietly past. Then the sound of the ferry would slowly get lower and lower. Only when the sound began to die did we know that it was moving away.

And that's what writing is like. You come as close to the bones of a thing as you can, but you know, you always know, that you rarely see the thing dead on. The truth of a person, a concept, even a memory can be that ferry in the fog. You get as close to it as you can, all the time hoping it doesn't run over you, but sometimes you never

Chapter 12. On Connection

quite see it and then you know you've gone beyond. You keep writing but you're only getting further away.

They say the truth can set you free, but it can also destroy what fragile coping you have. Better to figure out what dose you can live with. Unfortunately, as a writer that option is out. You have sworn, in some subterranean ritual, to tell the truth or you are not a writer. Writers hunt authenticity with a fervor that would match Larry Bird diving into the stands in search of a ball.

I don't understand connection, its subtle shades and blaring colors, the havoc that can result when people don't have the capacity for it, the ways in which its presence can enrich and its loss can poison your life. It is a shapeshifter, as fluid as water and as necessary for life. For me, it has always been the ferry in the fog.

Without it, most people wither like leaves cut off from a tree, but the Achilles' heel of love is loss. Anyone who has had someone very close to them die knows all too well the price of connection. So, what of the psychopathic offenders I see, who have no such attachments? Are they happier? Is life better if there are no strings attached? The odd thing is that without attachment, paranoia and callousness seem to fill the vacuum. Maybe—almost certainly—there are Zen monks out there who hold on to nothing, love no one in particular, and feel at peace, but that takes 10,000 hours of meditation just to get you in the ballpark. It is not intuitive or easily acquired. For ordinary people, lack of attachment leads to no peace at all. I don't see why it has to work this way. Care about no one and you become a marauding monster who can shoot a seven-months-pregnant woman because she has no drugs to rob. Care about someone and you are a hostage to fate—your chance of peace forever tied to their well-being, over which you have no control. Lose them and you have as much chance of cutting your losses as you do of gnawing off a phantom limb. Is there a third door?

I am often surprised at the intricacies of connection. Now you see it; now you don't. Even among violent offenders, I have sometimes been brought up short. Not every violent man is a psychopath.

I asked a gang banger with an impressive resume of criminal activity why he stayed in a business where prison or death were almost inevitable consequences. At first, the exchange was normal—well, normal is a relative term—at least, it was typical of other conversations I have had. He replied:

> It's not all bad. It's been financially lucrative. I be in the place where I can make decisions ...
>
> *Drug dealing?*
> A. That's in my history.
>
> *Robberies?*
> A. I don't do that. I have guys who do that. I'm too ambitious. Too charismatic. Too eloquent in my speech. That's for guys. Drugs are the same way. That's for guys who can't get it any other way. That's not for my status. That's a guaranteed trip to prison.
>
> Batteries as well. I've caught that in prison. I smashed two correctional guys, and I broke some bones, but I don't get in trouble for that kind of thing.... Since then, I haven't been no conduct reports for that.
>
> *Assaults on the street?*
> A. I don't do that. I have guys for that. I'm no longer in a position where I have to deal with that.... I've been off the street level since 22.
>
> *Are you saying you are on an administrative level?*
> A. That's why I have been admonished by the higher ups. They say, "You're an outstanding guy but you are impulsive."

I don't doubt he's high on the food chain in his gang, but I think he's just bragging when he talks about how eloquent he is, indulging in the usual grandiosity of offenders. But then I ask him about his relationships with women and he says:

> I don't play disloyal games. If I'm in a relationship, I'm in a relationship. I'd take loyalty over love any day.
>
> Love is an adjective; loyalty is a verb.
>
> Love has no boundaries. Or expectations or limitations. You can love someone and never say a word to them. But when you are loyal you have obligations, boundaries, expectations, and limitations. You can talk love. You can't talk loyalty. You gotta show it.

Chapter 12. On Connection

He stops me in my tracks. I am sitting seven steel doors from the green grass outside. I am talking with a man sitting shackled, a man who has done nothing that I respect and much that I despise, and yet he has said something about connection more eloquent and truer than anything I could say. In these interviews I hear a lot of counterfeit coins thrown on the table, but every once in a while, I hear the unmistakable ring of truth.

Before you get too misty-eyed, please remember that he had over 100 sex partners, and since he was pretty continuously in one relationship or another, it is extremely unlikely that all of these sex partners occurred between relationships. Sexual fidelity is probably not included in his definition of loyalty to his partners. In fact, he is likely far more loyal to his gang than to any mate or child of his. But still, I have learned something and understood something that I didn't know before he spoke.

His way of showing loyalty causes society a few problems. A few years ago, he claims that someone shot up his gang's drug house. What we know for sure is that he went over to that man's house, and despite seeing the man's children clearly through the window, he sprayed the house with bullets.

> A. He lost the fight. He wasn't arrested cause we didn't call the police. Then that night around midnight, we went over to his crib and shot it up.
>
> *Who else was there?*
> A. His kids, his lady. I saw them clearly through the window. I missed his kids by two or three inches. I was trying to kill all of them. There was no question about it.
>
> *Why were you trying to kill all of them? All of them didn't do anything to you.*
> A. I don't care about his kids, his mom, his wife.... If I cared about them, I wouldn't have shot his house.... I play for keeps.

He now says he has figured out he shouldn't have tried to shoot the kids. It is progress, but it took him a decade in prison before he even questioned whether there was anything wrong with shooting the kids. But whatever he is, and whatever his crimes, he does know something about connection. He understands loyalty, maybe in the same misguided way a Confederate soldier did. Loyalty runs like granite in the South and got us into that despicable war. People who never had the money to buy slaves and never would fought for the South, based solely on loyalty.

Later I score his psychopathy test. People high in psychopathy have little or no concern for others. They lack a conscience and are generally out only for themselves. Despite all the violence he has committed, he is not a psychopath. His conscience may be on life support, but it is there. But I could have told you that when he tutored me on love and loyalty.

We are a tribal species, a species for whom love and loyalty is first of all shown to family, then to intimates, and then to those who seem most like us. We are loyal to institutions with which we identify whether our high schools, our teams, or our country. That collides with our abstract sense of fairness, which says someone of another color or ethnic group or country of origin should have the same opportunity to get a job or move up the ladder as the person who is more like us, more like the person offering the job or making the decision. And of course, they should. But what we grandly call nepotism is nothing more than our tribal instincts asserting themselves. What we call implicit bias is nothing more than loyalty to kin—in the broadest sense. Of course, this isn't fair. It isn't fair that a white male will typically choose another white male over any female or a male of a different color, all the time telling himself the white male candidate is a better candidate, and it has nothing at all to do with bias. But what has fairness to do with biology? We're the only species that even pays lip service to fairness. The zebra has no recourse to the courts when the lion closes in. In the animal world, might always makes right. Lions stick with lions; zebras stick with zebras. Biology never embraced affirmative action.

Gang loyalty is no different than other kind of loyalty in its basic mechanism—no different than two high school teams squaring

Chapter 12. On Connection

off—except for the addition of high-powered weapons. Those in the gang are "us," and those across town doing the very same thing within the same structure are "them." When we complain of sexism and racism—and I frequently and fervently complain—we forget how rich the NFL is on the same basic mechanism—loyalty to one group over another. We sit in giant stadiums on Sundays and watch players make tens of millions of dollars and owners hundreds of millions and we think the dyadic aggression we see, the sum-loss game, the I-am-on-one-side-and-you-are-on-the-other is harmless. We are *loyal* to our team, and don't think it has anything to do with losing a promotion on Monday because a white male chose another white male who was, deep in his subconscious, on his team. That's implicit sexism or racism, and this is sports. Sports are fun! Sexism and racism are bad! But it is all tribalism, pure and simple, and it works well in sports and video games, and pretty badly, nearly everywhere else.

Antisocial offenders can be fully capable of loyalty—to their neighborhoods or their families or their gangs or their sports teams. They're just not loyal to us, to the larger social system. But psychopaths are different. Psychopaths are not loyal to anyone or anything. They are equal opportunity betrayers. They will snitch on another gang member as readily as a gang rival. They never made the leap from advancing and protecting their own interests to doing the same for others close to them. They stand outside the social contract the rest of us join without even knowing it. But while the lack of connection, of love and loyalty, may make them impervious to loss, it does not seem to nourish them, enrich them, create room inside them. It seems to put them constantly on red alert, in full battle dress, ready to go to war over a plumber not knocking on the screen door. There is no joy without connection, the price be damned.

Chapter 13

On Being Safe: Guns and Poses

I go to yoga, eat vegan and meditate. My entire career has been in the service of reducing violence. If I could, I would eliminate guns from the face of the planet. I support every gun law ever written and many that haven't been. I am all too aware that in addition to a professional criminal class who favors firearms, we have a large group of unstable "normal" citizens who cannot cope with their lives and think shooting people in a movie theater or a mall will make them feel better. Somehow dying by suicide after taking out a classroom of kids is going out with glory. In some ways they are more dangerous than professional criminals as the latter are motivated by profit. Criminals are at least as likely to try to sell you drugs as they are to mug you for your wallet. There is no profit to be made in mall shootings, and thus they are frowned on by the professional criminal. It is the irrational, ticking time bomb of hate in the unstable group of Americans who walk into their offices one morning with a semi-automatic that frightens me most.

While there are numerous sane gun owners, I don't personally think their right to own a gun outweighs my right not to be shot while watching *Batman*. All in all, we'd all be better off without guns, but the NRA (the first two letters stand for Not Rational …) seems intent on making sure that every unstable individual in the country can legally own a semi-automatic assault rifle that would take down the Russian army before police have time to arrive. If I ever put a bumper sticker on my car, it will be "If it weren't for the NRA, I wouldn't have to own a gun."

Chapter 13. On Being Safe: Guns and Poses

And that's the point. I do own one. Not to hunt. I would never shoot an animal. My 10-year-old neighbor had some issues to work through as a younger child and we have hung out together. He wrote an essay about me for class in which he described me as a "good person to talk to when your brain is full of weird thoughts." He also wrote, "She respects all people and all animals. Well, maybe not all people." He appears to know me well. I do respect all animals but not necessarily all people. I would find it a lot harder to shoot Bambi than Ted Bundy.

But put a gun in my hand, and I—like a lot of Americans—discover it feels right there. I am standing in a firing range in North Carolina looking at a Sig 320 9 mm. This is a truly modular firearm. Take it apart and screw on a different barrel and you have a different caliber. But I'm not staring at it with a look of pure sick puppy love because of its modular nature. I like the way it feels in my hand, the ease of the slide, the smooth and easy 5.5-pound trigger pull. The 12-pound trigger pull New York some police have to deal with or the slides that require weight training to rack are not for me.

Still, do I need another gun? No, I do not. I have a reliable Ruger snub-nosed .357 revolver, a gun that you can't screw up: no safety to turn off, no slide to pull. If it's loaded, you just pick it up and point it. It's a middle-of-the-night gun, a gun you can't forget how to use when the adrenaline hits. It's not that accurate at distances, but the only distance I would have to shoot someone at would be the length of a room. I put the .320 down. I'm just here to shoot a little. I'm not looking for a gun. But later, when I leave town, I can still feel the .320 pulling at me, like a man you turned down and aren't sure you should have.

I am a certified degree-holding, blue state feminist, and yet I, like a lot of Americans, have guns written into my DNA. All I can squeak out of my liberal leanings is that I disapprove of my love of guns: it makes no sense for anyone but a military professional to be so enamored. But I am, and we are, and that's the way it is.

I can't reconcile those two sides of me, the part that believes in self-protection and loves shooting guns and the part that knows the world would be better off if I and everyone else weren't allowed to own one. But then again, there are many things I can't reconcile, for example, justice and compassion.

Granted, my situation is a little different than most people's. The testimony I give and the reports I write regularly anger the kind of people who don't necessarily sue you when they get mad. They start cleaning their guns instead. Nonetheless, because of what I know about violence, it is a little confusing to me how *comfortable* I feel with a gun in my hand and how much safer I feel with one when camping alone in a remote area. But that's the problem. A lot of people feel comfortable with a gun in their hands—guns are fun to shoot—and level of confidence has nothing to do with level of skill or degree of rationality.

I am not a complete fool. I didn't just buy a gun, put bullets in it, and hope for the best. I have taken gun courses, I practice, and I am licensed to carry in 31 states. I study the laws of the states I will be passing through before taking a road trip to make sure I am in compliance. My gun is locked up at home, and most of the time when I travel it is in "transport" mode rather than "concealed carry" mode, i.e., it is empty, locked up, out of my reach as the driver with the ammunition in a separate part of the car. But despite the classes, the private lessons, and the practice, I don't fool myself that I have the kind of training that ensures I would respond well in an emergency. How would I know? I've never been in one.

Well, once, but that's before I had guns, and that's the reason I have them. There was a time when I didn't think I needed one or needed to be all that concerned about my personal safety. There was a time when I went off happily to work and dealt with violence and abuse on a daily basis, then came home and lived my life as though neither of those things could reach out and touch me personally.

In 1994 I was living in an isolated house in the countryside of New Hampshire with my two nine-month-old babies and entirely unconcerned with security. The house had two neighbors, both out

Chapter 13. On Being Safe: Guns and Poses

of sight and hearing, and the nearest state road was a half-mile away. The actual road to the house was an unpaved, private road the three houses maintained. Given the house was surrounded by trees my curtains were never closed: I didn't expect the deer to be too interested. Nor did I lock the doors. God forbid, someone who works with sex offenders every week should ever consider the possibility that one might stalk them.

Living in the country was the main reason I had moved to New Hampshire. I was recently out of graduate school, and while Cambridge was not the metropolis then that it is now, even so the Charles River had long ago lost all claim to being part of the natural world. It had moved permanently into the realm of the "precious"—the landscaped and manicured parks we pretend are nature. It's the difference between a styled poodle and a wolf.

"There are some who can live without wild things and some who cannot," Aldo Leopold wrote (Leopold, 1949). I have always felt half alive in towns and cities. I didn't want neighbors. I wanted deer who wandered through the yard. I wanted utter quiet. I wanted pitch-black nights where the stars looked so close together they could have been lights from a celestial city.

I had a new German Shepherd, and she began to bark constantly, obsessively almost every night. I had no idea anyone was out there, and the barking was so constant I thought she was barking at the inhabitants of the forest. I had infant twins at the time who were woken up by the barking. I ended up giving the dog away to someone looking for a Shepherd.

After that, I woke one night to the sound of a phone being knocked off a table in the living room and landing with a loud clatter. At that point I was working all day and feeding the twins all night and so chronically exhausted I was literally seeing double most nights. I didn't even get up. I thought the cat must have done it. It did cross my dazed and diminished brain that the cat was a pretty graceful girl and never knocked anything over. Maybe a poltergeist? You don't think straight when you're seeing double. An intruder? That didn't seem possible in idyllic New Hampshire. No one knew I lived there. Later I remembered that someone did.

The denial came to a screeching halt the day I came home and found all the windows open and both wood stoves blazing with fresh wood in them. It was winter and most certainly I had not left the windows so. Too, I knew the wood stoves could not have lasted 14 hours wide open. I called the local police attached to a nearby village. They came out but did not believe me. Nothing had been stolen. Why would anyone come in and not steal anything? Out of my hearing, they asked the nanny if I was making it up. She said no vehemently, but it made no impression. Maybe kids screwing around?

I wasn't satisfied and called a police officer I had worked with from another town. He had grown up hunting for food and knew the forests well. He came to the house and went searching through the woods. When he finished, he called me outside and said, "He's not a woodsman. He's parking on the logging trail and following the power lines to come in." The moment he said that I remembered one of the neighbors saying he had heard a car door slam on the logging trail in the middle of the night. We had both chalked it up to teenagers looking for a place to park. "Let me show you something," he went on. He took me a short distance from the house and showed me two vantage points on a little knoll in the woods closest to the house, one where you could see into the bathroom and the other into the bedroom. There was a path worn between them. I'm not sure what I did at that point. I think I sat down on the ground.

I started searching through my memory for which offenders I had worked with who were capable of getting in my house and might hold a grudge at a report I had written or testimony I had given. The list was depressingly long. Nor did it help to make it. It was impossible to accuse anyone without any evidence. As for me, I put the house on the market. I took a three-day gun course and I carried two babies and a .357 at the same time when going from the house to car and the car to the house until the house sold. When home, I locked the

Chapter 13. On Being Safe: Guns and Poses

doors and closed the windows. The house sold quickly, and I moved to town.

I would have gone on, never knowing the identity of the intruder were it not for serendipity. When I was in graduate school, I had a friend who was dating a cardiologist named David. Unfortunately, David had a psychotic break and became paranoid and obsessed with my friend. She eventually broke up with him, but before the relationship ended, he and my friend had come up to see me at the house I still lived in.

After the incident with the open windows and after I moved to town, my mentor from Harvard Graduate School, Sunny, went out on her front porch to pick up a newspaper. David was standing there in front of an old beat-up car. After greeting him, Sunny commented on the condition of his car. "Yes," he said, "I bought it from my father."

"David," she said gently, "your father has been dead for 20 years."

"Yes, I know," he said. "I bought it from my father's ghost. It's a terrible car, but what can you expect from my father's ghost? Where's Anna?" he added. "She's moved."

"I lost track of her years ago," Sunny said, went into the house, and called me.

How else could David have known that I had just moved unless he had been there recently? I called a police officer friend in Kenosha, Wisconsin, just to get her advice and discovered she already knew David. In the wildest of coincidences, he had come from that area and after his psychotic break had gone back there and driven a car up over the curb trying to kill several college students who were walking on the sidewalk. He claimed he could tell by just looking at them that they were gay and coming on to him. When police searched his car, they found writings on which states had the death penalty.

When my friend sent out a request for information over police channels, she found out that the FBI was very interested in David. They said he had been in several cities at the time men were murdered and dismembered with enough skill that they suspected the killer had medical training. They also said the Secret Service were interested as he had shown up on Martha's Vineyard when President Clinton was there. I was standing in my mentor's house when the FBI called her about the encounter with him. "Is he really dangerous?" she asked. It was hard for her to believe. There was a pause and the agent said, "Just don't turn your back on him."

David had never recovered from his mental illness, nor his obsession with my friend after she left him. He had been living off old friends and former girlfriends for years. He would make the circuit, going to one house and then another. Typically, his hosts would feel sorry for him and let him live there, but eventually they would have to ask him to leave. He would become aggressive, impossible to live with. While most of his stays were with the homeowner's permission, I was told that one couple came back from vacation and found him living in their basement. David had even called me and asked me if he could stay at one point, years earlier, shortly after his break-up with my friend. I knew he was irrational and aggressive, and I had said no. So, years later he came anyway, stalked me, violated my privacy, and eventually got into my house. Years after the fact, it is still uncomfortable to think that a psychotic man with aggressive tendencies whom police suspected was a serial killer was in my remote and isolated house while I, my nanny, and my babies slept.

I moved away from the country. I raised my babies with neighbors on each side, both in New Hampshire and later in Madison, Wisconsin. I left the deer and the dark nights. I kept a gun in the house. I also left any lingering illusion of safety. There are few things I have lost that I have missed more.

Chapter 14

The Social Contract

I moved to Madison when the babies were four. I moved because I was constantly triggered in New Hampshire by my son's death. Every street was a street I had driven down with him. He had gone to the only local school. Everyone knew of my loss. I had no privacy and no chance to escape, even for a moment, the legacy of his death. I wanted to choose who I told and who I didn't that I had lost a child. But most of all I did not want to raise the twins in the shadow of their brother's death.

I chose Madison, Wisconsin, because I had an opportunity to join a private practice and work with corrections. After I moved, I began to work with incarcerated inmates and later with civilly committed sex offenders. The incarcerated inmates I worked with came predominantly from a prison formerly called a supermax. The inmates had sued, saying that the fact the institution was called a "supermax" was prejudicial to their chances of getting jobs afterwards, etc. The name of the institution was changed but nothing else. The visits still had inmates in one room and visitors behind glass in another. The security was so tight that after the fence with razor wire there was a lethal electric fence. I questioned this, and the warden joked, "Don't worry, Anna, no inmate will ever get anywhere near that fence. We may fry a couple of maintenance men but no inmates." A state the size of Wisconsin did not need a supermax that could have contained every super violent offender in the Midwest, but the entire institution with its insane level of security had been built by a former governor who was known for his expansive opinion of himself and who wanted to do big projects, whether they were needed or not.

Wardens in any prison do not ask psychologists to evaluate inmates who are sane, well controlled, and reasonably compliant. There were inmates who had all three of those characteristics in the institution formerly known as a supermax, but I never saw them. I saw the white supremacist who went into black neighborhoods and killed "drug dealers." I evaluated the cartel member who ran drugs from Mexico and had gotten caught. I talked to the Chicago gangster who came up to the town of Superior to "cool off" after killing someone in Chicago and who ended up having the prosecutor's house firebombed by his gang after he was arrested for another murder in Superior. I interviewed a man who kidnapped his ex-wife, and after keeping her and his children for days, released the children and killed the woman. I evaluated the man who saw teenagers swimming from a bridge, got his rifle, and shot them for no reason at all. He said that afterward that he felt the most peace during the day after he did that than he had ever felt in his life. Most were not sex offenders but were violent psychopaths with no limits or inhibitions. Some were sadists who got a high from hurting others.

I also began to evaluate sex offenders in a neighboring state who were considered possible candidates for civil commitment, and later I began evaluating offenders who had already been committed to see if they were ready for release. It was here that I obtained experience with high-risk sex offenders. The criteria for being civilly committed as a sex offender was a history of committing sex offenses, a diagnosis that predisposed the offender to committing future sexually violent offenses (for example, pedophilia), and a probability of reoffending that was "more likely than not."

These folks were not like the outpatients I had previously treated. The outpatients had histories of child molestation or rape but not *histories* of child molestation and/or rape. The men in the prison formerly known as a supermax and the civil commitment program in a neighboring state had scores of victims and as many as 10 previous convictions whereas outpatient offenders tended to have one or two known victims and/or convictions. The ones in prison I was asked to

Chapter 14. The Social Contract

see typically had a level of callousness unmatched by anything I had seen doing outpatient therapy. The patients who were civilly committed were either callous or so deviantly attracted to children or sadism that they were unable to control it.

With parenting my first son, I was laissez faire, thinking he could figure most things out on his own. After his loss, I became a helicopter parent with my twins, supervising everything to the nth degree. I also had worked with enough offenders at that point that I didn't trust anyone all that much. I signed up to be the parent representative for so many sports groups that when my children were in high school and the baseball coach asked the kids whose mother might be a parent representative, five boys raised their hands and suggested me. I learned to score baseball, so I had an excuse for hanging around the Little League team. This culminated in a year I helped coach Little League. Ph.D.s were common in Madison with its giant university, and one night the three coaches for our team realized we all had them. One of the coaches shook his head and said, "It's a wonder these kids have won a single game."

There is no small amount of emotional whiplash in going from T-ball games to torture. I put up such a wall between the two that I couldn't remember anything from work at home, and if I did, I quickly learned no one wanted to hear it, no matter how sanitized, anonymous, and generic a story was. It was a double life but on both ends it was a life of purpose, and I thought my dad would understand a life of purpose.

* * *

"If there's a riot," the warden said, "it'll start right here." My work with corrections had taken me into the heart of a maximum-security prison. I looked around at the clattering printing presses and the inmates busy working them. None of them acknowledged our presence which, in itself, was a little eerie, since it was obvious every single inmate in the warehouse space knew the warden was there. My first thought was, "Then why don't we just mosey along?" It was 1997 and I was new to corrections, having worked with outpatient offenders and victims for most of my career. Safety of one sort or another was often on my mind. Hanging around the one spot in the prison that the warden thought was the most dangerous—with no guards around—struck my beginner's mind as less than prudent.

Not wanting to sound like a wimp, I said instead, "Why here?"

"Because most of the men in this room are lifers, and there are a lot of them." And this, of course, is the other side of the death penalty. Lifers have very little to lose in a non-death penalty state such as Wisconsin. What are we going to do to them? Give them another life sentence? Of course, segregation can always be used as a consequence, but many inmates are immune to it, and a few prefer it—those without people skills, those afraid of other inmates, and those who are habituated to it.

He sauntered across the room to the door, and we stepped outside. "I was walking right along this route," he said, going back to the main topic of our tour. "I was heading toward the main building. Fred was walking with me. He was a social worker here. It was a picnic day when families were allowed to come in and have a picnic with their inmate. I heard footsteps running behind me, but I didn't turn."

"Why not?" I asked.

"Because if it was something, I wanted to protect my chest."

I mulled this over, but it didn't make a lot of sense to me. You can fight back a lot better if you can see your attacker, and you can get to the heart from front or back, but I didn't say anything. I wasn't there.

"He came over my shoulder," he said, "just like this," and he demonstrated, an imaginary shiv in his hand. I noticed he was suddenly tense. I was aware that he has PTSD from the assault, and you could see it beginning to come out. He was not so much describing what happened as reliving it. They ended up on the ground with him on his back and the attacker over him with the shiv. "And here's the thing. I had this medallion I had bought just a few days ago." He stopped at the spot of the attack and looked around. "I bought it from a shop selling Indian jewelry. Something just told me to buy it. And

Chapter 14. The Social Contract

the shiv hit the medallion. That's the only reason he didn't stab me in the chest. This little medallion," he says, showing me a small piece of metal about the size of a 50-cent piece. I marveled at this part of the story. I could never put it in a mystery. Who would believe it? There is a limit on how fantastic the story can be in fiction; in life there is no limit.

The inmate got the shiv above the warden's eye. For a long moment he and the warden arm wrestled over whether the shiv was going in the warden's eye while the social worker was on the inmate's back trying to pull him off. Then the guards were there grabbing the inmate and it was over.

The attack was taped from the towers, and later I watched the grainy footage. All the time the attack was occurring the other inmates in the yard were glancing from the fighting men to the towers, from the towers to the fighting men. The warden believed that without armed men in the towers, other inmates would have gotten involved to his detriment. I wondered if they weren't simply looking to see if the guards were going to shoot someone, but they couldn't—not without hitting the warden.

Fast forward 17 years to 2014 and I am in a room with Gonzales,[1] the man with the shiv that day. He is sitting in a chair bolted to the floor, and his wrists and legs are shackled to a chain that leads to a bolt in the floor. He is still on administrative confinement which is, essentially, segregation and means he can't meet with anyone alone without being shackled and two guards outside the door. This particular door even has a window in it. Administrative confinement is similar to segregation but with a few more privileges. It is for inmates who have served their segregation time but are judged too dangerous to go back into general population. Gonzales has been in segregation or administrative confinement since the attack on the warden. No one has any idea if he is still dangerous. There's no easy way to tell except to turn him loose in the general population and see if he kills someone. Given his history, corrections has been reluctant to do that.

Gonzales has complained he has a "PCP-like psychosis" from his suntan lotion, and I am interviewing him for an evaluation:

Aren't you in your cell almost 23 hours a day?
    A. Yes.

Q. Why exactly do you need suntan lotion?
    A. They sell it in canteen, and I use it on my face because my face gets dry.

For a moment the situation seems surreal. I am in a maximum security prison talking with a leader of the Spanish Cobras who is guilty, not only of the attack on the warden, but whose initial, admitting offense was robbing a man and then shooting him three times in the face and once in the heart, and, in addition, who was one of the leaders of the worst prison riot in the state's history, a riot in which 14 staff members were taken hostage in 1983, *and we are discussing moisturizers.*

The prison doctor has his doubts that the suntan lotion has anything to do with how the inmate is feeling but made the practical suggestion that he quit using it. Nonetheless, the inmate is upset about his recent "psychosis" and wants an evaluation.

I start with my standard spiel. I am a psychologist and consultant for the Department of Corrections (DOC). I do evaluations of inmates in different prisons when DOC requests one. "Oh," he interrupts me, "you're a gunslinger."

"I guess," I say. "In a way." No one else has ever framed what I do quite that way. I have been called everything from "lunatic" to "war horse" to "princess of darkness" to even "Jackie Robinson"[2]—but never gunslinger. Still, he sees things in terms of gun fights. I tell him the interview is voluntary, that he can terminate it at any point, that he can refuse to answer any questions he doesn't want to answer, that he can tell me anything he thinks is relevant that I don't think to ask, and that he can ask me any questions about the process that he wishes. I tell him I will write a report and that the report will go into his Psychological Services Unit (PSU) file. I tell him the interview

Chapter 14. The Social Contract

is not confidential: anything he says to me can go into the report. I also tell him that I am using a computer because I have my interview on it and I ask him the same things I ask everyone else. Finally, I tell him that I type his answers to avoid misquoting him by relying on my memory or on scribbled notes. Surprisingly many inmates with a history of suspiciousness and paranoia like Mr. Gonzales don't mind the computer. They want to avoid being misquoted also. Gonzales doesn't object.

I ask him what he means by a "PCP-like psychosis." He is certainly not psychotic now, and none of the notes by PSU or others documented any sort of psychotic symptoms.

> I felt like I was tranquillized. Also, that wall of inhibition collapsed. I was saying things I don't ordinarily say. I keep to myself. I was snapping to people. I ... I am very courteous. I got to arguing with guys.... I got to snapping on them.

Certainly, that would be a change. Gonzales has a multi-decade track record—long before the attack on the warden—of keeping himself under absolutely tight control. He almost never spoke to staff or anyone else who wasn't in his gang. Courteous might be a stretch, at least to staff, but he certainly wasn't known for emotional displays.

"Is there a possibility you are changing?" I ask. After all, Gonzales is now 57. Most anti-social offenders reduce their anti-social behavior as they age and it is possible that some psychopaths do also. Gonzales dismisses that idea. He has always been the same:

> One thing I try to do is try not to be a reflection of this institutional madness. Segregation causes the façade to peel back for some people, and you see people for who they really are. And you see the evil....
>
> I found myself like guys told me, "You don't fit in. You don't fit in with that criminal mentality. You don't fit in with the foul nature of a lot of guys."

It may surprise the reader that someone with Mr. Gonzales's track record, not just of attacking a high-ranking prison official, but also with a long-standing history of gang violence and murder, might not see himself as having any of the qualities associated with the term "evil"—in fact, not see himself as even having a criminal mentality. But I have discovered that most of the offenders I see, even those who made their entire living by crime, those who have track records of gang violence, personal violence, institutional violence, and even torture, do not see themselves as criminals. They do admit to "breaking the law" with great regularity, however. He goes on:

> I felt like the same symptoms of PCP. I felt like I was high on dope.... I took it a couple of times, but I didn't care for the high.... It had me arguing with these guys. I'm not an argumentative type of guy. I'm an introvert. I came out of my shell.

It appears that Mr. Gonzales is so unused to having feelings that, when he started having them, he thought he was psychotic. He is also upset at what he sees as a drop in his habitual hyper-vigilance and grudge-bearing:

> It's hard for me to point out. Like guys disrespecting me through my PCP psychosis and they asked me for something, and I gave it to him. People say, "This guy disrespected you. What are you doing?" I forgot he just said it.

I go through a careful mental status exam to be sure, but I can't find any evidence of psychosis, either present or in his description of the past. He had some anxiety, but no racing thoughts, no delusions, no hallucinations, no thought disorder, no symptoms of mania, no depression. Nor were any reported by anyone who interacted with him at the time. I don't think he's playing me either, as it is totally out of character for him. He has a very long history of hostility to staff, to say the least, but none of seduction and manipulation.

What is wrong with Mr. Gonzales isn't on the psychotic side of things but on the personality disorder side. He has the unholy trilogy of paranoia, suspiciousness, and grievance-based thinking that I find in almost every violent offender. The grievance is clear.

Chapter 14. The Social Contract

Why did you attack a warden?
   A. Overwhelming rage. The pain. When my brother Robert committed suicide, he wouldn't let me go to the wake. That was being vindictive because of my other case [the riot].

Although I should know better, I am astonished he took that personally. I ask him if he can see it from any other point of view. If he were a warden, could he let a high-ranking gang member go to a wake which would be heavily attended by gang members—not to mention if that gang member had been a leader in the worst prison riot in state history and not to mention that the gang member was in for murder? He'd be crucified if he sent two officers in harm's way like that. It's obvious to me that no warden could clear that. Gonzales doesn't see it that way. No, he insists. It was retaliation for the riot. He mentions that the warden was once on the staff at the prison where the riot occurred. It was because of that, he says, that he wouldn't let Mr. Gonzales go. Mr. Gonzales considers himself entitled. Policies and procedures don't apply to him. If someone prevents Mr. Gonzales from doing something he wants to do, it is personal and a sign of disrespect.

Let's go back a step. How did Gonzales get where he is? This is not going to be the usual diatribe about poverty and abuse, which sounds more to my ear like an excuse for violence. Let's talk about specific connections. How did Gonzales learn to despise authority in all forms and take every single rule and regulation as a personal affront?

Let's start with you. Where did you learn to respect authority? No doubt you learned to respect authority from your parents. It began, perhaps, when you picked up the fire truck to hit your brother in the head and someone much larger than you took it out of your hand and said "no" in a convincing voice, possibly accompanied by a swat. Still, the "no" itself would have been sufficient. And here already the track diverges.

If the person who said "no" is even vaguely reasonable, is a "good enough" parent, as the psychiatrist and pioneer in temperament studies Stella Chess, used to say, then you will accept the "no" and eventually modify your behavior when an authority figure isn't standing over you. This is your first lesson that violence is not OK. Of course, accepting the "no" presupposes you are being fed, that the person in charge provides a modicum of interpersonal warmth, that you do not come to feel you are in the presence of someone who means to do you harm, the malevolent transformation that Harry Stack Sullivan described. You're a long way from the *concept* of authority, but you are paying attention: someone you love is telling you "no" and they are big enough to enforce it. Since you'd rather be praised than yelled at, you get with the program.

In school, whether day care, preschool, or grammar school, your next authority figures were teachers. You can survive an arbitrary teacher or two as long as most teachers are generally reasonable. They become authority figures and now you are getting the gist of it: big people—your parents, friends' parents, and teachers—they're in a class by themselves. No one says to you in second grade, "These are authority figures," but you understand: you have to listen to them, and by then, using a phone cord to strangle a teacher is pretty much out of the question.[3] Still, size plays a big role, and small children tend to do what any adult says—which makes it very hard to get kids to obey some adults and not others, e.g., family and acquaintances who want to molest them.

Then there may be coaches or ministers or priests, and in adolescence, the Piagetian bell of abstract thinking goes off and the *concept* of authority figures becomes clear. By adulthood you will pull over for a police officer you have never seen before, take your clothes off and spread your legs for a man you have never met if he's called a doctor, quake if a person with IRS credentials shows up at your door—even if your taxes are prepared by the world's most obsessive accountant. You have the concept of roles and, more specifically, the concept of one particular role—*authority figure*—and your first response on meeting one is acceptance and acquiescence, not aggression. Your default mode is deference, and it takes something—a

Chapter 14. The Social Contract

police officer slamming your face in the road for jaywalking, for example—before you even think of rebelling. And even then, you see that particular person as an exception to the notion that most authority is reasonable.[4]

Welcome to the social contract, the invisible set of rules and rights and regulations that really govern society. Sure, there are written laws with concrete penalties, but mostly we police ourselves. In addition there are social norms we obey which aren't written into laws. You don't walk into work and say to a colleague, "Good morning, you son of a bitch," even if you intensely dislike the person. Social norms say you are polite to coworkers. This is how I end up at a stoplight in the middle of the night in Wyoming, 50 miles from anywhere with no cars anywhere in sight, and yet I sat patiently waiting for a red light to turn green. I have done it so long it just seems natural to wait at a red light—even when I won't get caught and there's no point in sitting there waiting. Mostly, we obey the laws and only fiddle with those laws that have minimal consequences and social acceptance of fiddling—e.g., marijuana in states where it still isn't legal.

But Gonzales didn't grow up like that. The Gonzaleses of the world, the ones in my world, often had a crack dealer for a mother or father. Parents and/or boyfriends beat him with everything from coat hangers to electric cords to paddles to two-by-fours. No one said "sorry" later, and no one said they loved him. Some parents didn't necessarily beat their children but ignored them and neglected them. Learning to open a can as a young preschooler can be a life-saving skill.

I don't mean to imply that all criminals come from that kind of dysfunction and cruelty. Some psychopaths come from perfectly normal families—particularly those that were adopted: psychopathy is now thought to have a genetic component. But for many criminals, upbringing was at least a part of it. What they learned from their first authority figure was that authority is arbitrary, unfair, and violent to the point of being life-threatening. It was a matter of survival to resist it.

By the time school came, anyone who tried to control them was a target. They were socialized into violence as a way to solve problems, and they saw no way to understand the namby-pamby teachers who kept telling them to sit down and do their schoolwork. They resist, as they always have, but this time the consequences are different. Resisting a parent who is trying to kill you with a butcher knife or waving a gun around is one thing; resisting a teacher who is trying to teach you is another—but it doesn't seem like it is. Programmed that fear and respect are the same thing, you set about trying to establish yourself as the meanest *&^%$#@ in the classroom, sending another kid for stitches just to make a point. After all, you are *sure* he called you a name under his breath.

By adolescence, the Gonzaleses of the world have their own concept of authority. Authority is inherently unfair and arbitrary. People are out to get them. Anyone who wants to have power over them is an enemy. The only protection out there lies in people fearing them too much to mess with them, and that is as true of cops as it is of other drug dealers on the street. They begin to obsess and ruminate on retaliation for the slights and injuries that occur in everyday life. They think about them all day long. Insults, signs of disrespect become the lens through which they view the world. It is what they expect to see, and they are hypervigilant for interactions that convey "disrespect" each and every day. Nor do these slights have to be extreme. One morning in prison their food is cold. It is deliberate. Another day a guard smiles when she hands them a tray. She must have spit in it. Anyone who laughs talking to someone down the hall must be making fun of them. These are all real examples. Neutral acts become mini acts of aggression. Acts of kindness are not even noticed or are viewed with suspicion. Everyone is out for number one. Why would anyone do something for you unless they were making some kind of play, unless they wanted something?[5] In order to protect themselves they scan for offense, and because that is all they are looking for, that's all they see. On the inventories I give offenders when I interview them, the one item that almost all violent offenders

Chapter 14. The Social Contract

endorse is "I am suspicious of overly friendly strangers." They are suspicious of "overly friendly" acquaintances, family, and friends too. Perhaps all of us are a *little* suspicious of overly friendly strangers, but most of us entertain the possibility that they *might* be genuine. That is not a possibility if you live in Gonzales's world.

For most offenders that I interview, there is a kind of relief in having someone interested in the narrative of their lives. They don't typically come from environments where people were interested in them, even as children. For those that do, the offenders themselves usually blocked communication, as they were rebellious at an early age. Prison psychologists have their hands full with crisis management, and no prison I have ever been worked at has had the resources to provide regular one-on-one therapy. Even though I am only assessing them, it is still a chance to talk and put things together. For some, it is the only time someone has sat for hours and just listened.

But to accept the invitation to think about their lives, histories, motivations, and future plans requires a modicum of trust—not a huge amount, just enough not to think I am part of some large conspiracy designed to hurt them. Gonzales doesn't have it. He refuses a second session to finish up my evaluation. He said more than he meant to say in the first one. The paranoia surfaces and takes over like a parasite he had beaten back for a few minutes. He decides I was just trying to get information out of him about his offenses—although how talking about them can hurt him at this point, I have no idea.

He takes out an ethics complaint on me, saying I was supposed to be doing an evaluation of his PCP psychosis and I should never have asked him questions about his offenses. I respond by sending info about my protocol, about the fact the interview was voluntary, that he was told he could refuse to answer any questions he didn't want to answer, and that he could terminate the interview at any point. I send in my interview which I told him from the start I use with everyone. The complaint goes nowhere. But no doubt he is still ruminating about how I am going to use that information against him, and it fattens up the parasite of bitterness infesting his brain.

There is a large and interesting movement today to be kind to offenders, to treat them better, to rehabilitate them by helping them learn skills. I treat every single person I interview respectfully, but I am not naïve enough to think that respect or kindness or skill training alone will turn the tide of malevolence in a violent offender that was built up through a lifetime of training in harboring grudges. It's going to be more complicated than that.

≈ CHAPTER 15 ≈

Homes and Houses

The sailboat my second husband and I bought as graduate students was as light as a 25-foot empty Clorox bottle. With not enough headroom to stand up below and an aversion to heavy weather, it was not built for cruising. It was, as Mary White's father wrote in his famous essay "The Death of Mary White" (May 17, 1921, Kansas Historical Society), "as full of faults as an old shoe." We loved it anyway and sailed it up and down the New England coast relentlessly, good weather and bad. We spent most of our time off the coast of Massachusetts where it was moored, but it was Maine I loved best. With 5000 miles of coastline, there were far more harbors than sailboats. Unlike the Massachusetts coast where you would have to find a harbor for the night early or risk being crowded out, you could always find a cove in Maine where there might (or might not) be one other sailboat on the pristine water. There were lobstermen in every cove, and we would row our dingy up to one to buy a lobster for dinner, then sit on the back of our tiny boat with a glass of wine, watching a tired sun, like a sleepy toddler, lose its fight to stay up all night. It was home.

I've been thinking of home lately and what makes a house a home and what doesn't. By house, I mean any dwelling that people inhabit from igloos to tenement apartments to yurts to mansions: any place where humans dwell. A house is potentially a home but there are far more inhabited houses than homes. So, what makes a home? The offenders I see lived in dwellings, but few ever had a home.

Alain de Bouton wrote, "We need a home in the psychological sense as much as we need one in the physical: to compensate for a vulnerability. We need a refuge to shore up our states of mind, because so much of the world is opposed to our allegiances" (De Botton, 2006). Home is a refuge; it is solace, or it isn't a home. That is the one flat requirement that cannot be negotiated. No amount of remodeling or adding on rooms will change it. A home is safe. It is not a place where people live in fear, especially of other inhabitants. A home is incompatible with violence or belittling. Houses where nervous women wait for hostile/raging footsteps is not a home. A place where children cover their ears or turn up their video games to avoid hearing thudding sounds or screams from the floor below is not a home.

I work with violent sex offenders, and I am not one to think a grown man who rapes children should be given a break because he had a bad childhood. Even so, the childhoods of some of these men would make a statue weep: five-year-olds who ran away to live on the streets because it was safer than living at home. Children with crack-addicted mothers who ran drugs out of their homes and were too impaired to stop whatever man felt like raping their child. Fathers who alternated between brutality and indifference. Children who were starved. Children whose mothers came home from work and locked themselves in their rooms for the night with beer, potato chips and the TV, leaving the kids to find some cans and a can opener. "No one leaves home," Warren Shire wrote, "unless home is the mouth of a shark" (Shire, 2015). But sometimes your dwelling is the mouth of a shark. This is not just a problem of the poor any more than violence is. I remember a woman whose wealthy parents never ate with her—or had anything much to do with her, except her famous father when he was raping her. When the nanny was fired, the child's first thought was that she'd never eat again. The problem was solved, however. Her parents sent her to a restaurant every night in a taxi with a credit card, an eight-year-old sitting by herself and ordering dinner. Her house was a grand old building, but it was not a home.

There is a certain exclusivity to a home. The people who live there control who comes and goes. If there is no exclusivity, it is a

Chapter 15. Homes and Houses

public space. Often the men I see had families who blurred the boundaries. Not everyone could come in—police weren't welcome—but there was a steady stream of relatives and "friends," the latter being loosely defined. "Friends" were sometimes people the adults had partied with the night before who were too drunk or stoned to leave. "Friends" could be drug buyers, a variety of unknown men and women—the men almost always carrying weapons—whose solace came from chemicals. Often the adults told someone they had just met that they could live there. Strangers came and went, some living there for a few months and moving on. Paramours came and went. Female paramours could be dangerous to the children, but it was more often the mother's boyfriends whom the adult criminals I meet still don't want to talk about.

People have rights in their own home that they have nowhere else. For homeowners, the right to impact the property is extreme. They can build, remodel, and even demolish, needing only the occasional agreement of a zoning board or an HOA. Even for renters, the rights are extensive. The apartment owner can't simply walk in. Renters have a right to privacy, to live life as they choose. Community standards of behavior mostly don't apply in a home. There is such a thing as public drunkenness—which can land you in jail—but no legal admonition against private drunkenness. There is public misconduct but not private. Walk around nude in public and you will find yourself in jail, labeled a sex offender. Walk around nude in your home, and—depending on who's there or whether the curtains are closed—you may not have a problem. We are all required to conform our behavior to reasonable community standards in public but not in our own homes. Of course, we are supposed to follow the law. Child abuse is illegal in both public and private spaces. But who is to know? The right to privacy covers a multitude of crimes. Sherlock Holmes said: "You look at these scattered houses, and you are impressed by their beauty. I look at them, and the only thought which comes to me is a feeling of their isolation and of the impunity with which crime may be committed there" (Conan Doyle, 1892).

He held a rather negative view of privacy and the countryside but too often an accurate one of privacy, at least. Most of us do not require observers to keep us from abusing our children or our spouses, but some do. And that is the double-edged sword of privacy. Most enjoy it, but some misuse it. Without the strictures and constant oversight of others, the crimes that occur in private dwellings are far more difficult to detect. Homes require self-control over behavior. What separates a house from a home is whether the inhabitants have it. For some, the only controls are external. The buildings they dwell in are not homes. For many of us, homelessness strikes us as the ultimate horror, and it is a horror, but maybe not the ultimate one. There is a limit to how much abuse you can inflict in public.

A home has a certain aesthetic. By that, I don't mean anything to do with money. I have seen mansions where each room screamed "interior decorator" and were about as personal as the sales floor of a furniture store, albeit an expensive one. There was no sense of home. I have also seen a home where the occupant couldn't afford a vacuum cleaner, but the Walmart rug was brushed every day. Yes, cleanliness and order are part of it, although this rule is not as fixed as the one above. There have been times I have been in hippy homes where the emphasis on either cleanliness or order was not pronounced and yet the sunlight flowed through brightly-colored, window-covering cloths, landing on a brass incense burner or a hand-painted coffee cup. Such rooms glowed from reflected light. Some have an eye for beauty. A full artist's eye is by no means a requirement or most of us would not have homes, but there has to be some sort of care taken. It is the sense of care, the sense that someone notices this space, that someone loves it or the people in it enough to take care. And that is why the Walmart rug was as good as an Oriental in fostering a sense of home. It was loved, cared for.

A home must have life, and while one person can make a home, it is easier if there are other critters involved. I live alone and love it, but would I love it so much if two cats and a dog didn't stretch out before the fire? I don't think so. Walk in a house that has a cat or dog

Chapter 15. Homes and Houses

or pigeon or aardvark as a co-inhabitant and you are coming home to someone. I favor cats over aardvarks. A like-minded soul, Jean Cocteau, wrote, "I love cats because I enjoy my home; and little by little, they become its visible soul." Still, I grant that those who favor aardvarks can be at home. There are those talented enough to make a home with a fire and music and good books or art, but for me, buddies have always been essential. They just don't have to be human. These days, I prefer they aren't. I see plenty of humans during the day and enjoy their company, but at night I want to come home to quiet spaces where I can dance like nobody's watching, because nobody is.

Strange places are not home. A home is familiar, although some places are instantly familiar. Peter Hillary, St. Edmund Hillary's explorer son, wrote about his first experience in a tent, where he felt immediately that he was home from the first time he slept in one. Tents were part of his genetic code: he was born to them, so to speak. Once I learned to scuba dive well enough that I was not constantly scanning the instruments, I realized I was home. I was 70 feet below the surface in a world alien to everything on land, and yet I felt I belonged there. When I am on a diving vacation, the time between dives begins to really feel like a surface interval and my real life is underwater. Still, I grew up on the coast of North Carolina with, literally, the water in the front yard. As a child, I spent every possible moment sailing and water skiing. I am "water-wise," as the saying goes. Finding a way to breathe underwater just took away a frustrating barrier. So maybe for me, 70 feet below is just an extension, a new room in a home with which I was already familiar.

But for most of us, our houses gradually turn into homes. We don't fall in love instantly. It takes coming home, over and over again. It takes loving people in those spaces. It takes memories to turn a house into a home. Homes are not born full form when the moving truck leaves or when the boxes are finally unpacked. Houses are built, but homes are grown.

There is love somewhere in a home. Somebody has to love something or someone in that home. It isn't furniture for most people, but

I do love a table made out of a half cross-section of a giant redwood tree, once owned by a friend who died. But then I loved the friend too. I also love a hand-carved square-rigger sailing ship, exquisitely crafted by my grandfather in the early 1900s when, as a young man, he spent seven years in a rest home for people with TB. That was the only treatment back then: quarantine and rest. He met a sailor in the home who suggested he carve a square-rigger. A skillful carver, he said he didn't know how to rig it. The sailor told my grandfather if he could carve it, the sailor could rig it. My grandfather had seen plenty of square riggers sailing up and down the coast near his North Carolina home. He could carve it. The lines are taut today, a hundred years later. I remember touching the sails as a small child and drawing my hand back in surprise when I realized they were made of wood. They billowed so convincingly I thought they were canvas. "How did you do that?" I asked in wonder. He replied, "I don't mean to give you a short answer, honey, but it's all in the knowing how." Loved objects have stories and people attached to them. Take everything else but leave me my table and my sailboat, and I would have the beginnings of a home.

All of this is to say that a home is a physical manifestation of a psychological state. It is a projection outward of the world within. When we are young, homes produce psychological states of well-being and peace. To be able to create a home as an adult requires that we have internalized those states and projected them outward once again. Most phenomena tend to be spirals or waves and this inner/outer dynamic is surely a spiral. Have enough sense of safety in your own head to establish a home and the sense of repose you will gain in that space will create a greater sense of safety in your head and the spiral goes on.

But what happens when the only internal states in childhood are anxiety, anger, and fear? What of those who have never known a home and never known what it is like to have a place of repose where they feel safe. They often do badly in establishing homes. At worst they dwell in houses that feel as unsafe as the ones they grew

Chapter 15. Homes and Houses

up in. How do you establish a place of safety if you don't know what safety feels like? When I treat victims, I often start with imagining a safe place. I wrote earlier of the victims who do not know what I am talking about when I ask them to imagine a safe place and I am reduced to asking, "Well, can you imagine any place where you feel a little less afraid?"

People who establish real homes are not so quick to move. It takes a reason, a good reason, to pull up stakes and start growing a home somewhere else. A home has weight, gravitas, a magnetic pull. It is loved. A home is not something that can be easily re-established. It will take time and effort far beyond the moving. The offenders I have worked with often had families who moved multiple times a year. With nothing emotionally invested, there was nothing to hold them; one building was as good as another. Of course, moving several times a year, every year, is disastrous for children. They are forever strangers in every school they attend. The friendships they develop are fleeting, too short to be more than pencil marks on the heart, erased on the next stop down the line. Research has repeatedly shown that a relationship with a caring, prosocial adult outside the home can make the difference for children raised in adverse circumstances but constant moving means that relationships with teachers or coaches can gain no purchase. Hostility to authority ensures that such figures are met with defiance—no prior experience required. Brevity ensures there is not enough time to build a relationship that would compete with such preconceived notions.

It is possible I sell some such families short. Moving may not always be a sign of indifference. It may be that for some families, at least, the moving may not be the restlessness of nomads but a sign that the last dwelling, the last town, the last job fell short and moving is a sign of hope. Maya Angelou wrote, "The ache for home lives in all of us, the safe place where we can go as we are and not be questioned" (Angelou, 1991). Perhaps that ache drives some people onward, as though the next town will be home. And of course, there are military families who move in an organized system. But it is failure, not hope or a job requirement, that drives some abusive parents restlessly from place to place. The last job was lost because they showed up once too often drunk or stoned or didn't show up at all. The last housing was lost because they didn't pay the rent.

George Valliant argues that more people than you think overcome bad childhoods to be adults full of peace and purpose who create safe homes for themselves and others. Of course, he's right. People can learn. But the point is, people who grew up in houses but not homes have to learn something they never experienced. They have to create something they never had, which is a job in itself. When my daughter was in college, she gave me a potholder that said, "Home is where your mother is." It delighted me because home was never where my mother was. Indeed, I spent most of my childhood fantasizing about how wonderful it would be if my parents divorced and my mother left. My naïve childhood brain never considered the judicial system would have placed us with our mother and it was my father who would have left. Had I known that the prayers would have been to make the marriage last. Despite my loving father with whom I did feel safe, I didn't grow up in a home. She was always there, screaming, slapping, belittling, and carrying on. My first home was a silent gym. It took decades before I had enough repose in my head to bring that feeling of the silent gym into a real home. For others, there will never be enough decades.

When I ask friends and family what makes a home, the most common answer I receive is that a home is where you feel comfortable. But most of us feel comfortable in a variety of places: on vacation, at our friends' homes, even at work. Home is comfortable, but a kind of comfortable that eludes description. It is a place where everything feels familiar, where the space inside our heads takes visible form, a place the dweller has defined, where our internal world is manifest in color and line and form. Unless there is abject and total poverty, there are still choices, and those personal choices define the space. The door is the dividing line between the "real world" outside and the private world inside. It is the place where we are least

Chapter 15. Homes and Houses

on guard, least conscious of how others see us, least concerned with whether our words and actions conform to someone else's judgement. It elicits a kind of peace, or it is not a home. We do not often make distinctions between houses and homes, but we should. We simply say "homeless or not homeless," but really we mean housed or not housed. Our most violent citizens have mostly grown up homeless, regardless of how many houses they lived in.

Chapter 16

Hope

If all the sex offenders in the civil commitment program where I work were cars, they would be cars that have been wrecked time and time again. Worse, they would not be the cars that were run into; they would be the cars that did the running into. They would be the cars that T-boned another car carrying a mother and small child. There is no getting around the fact that high-risk, repeat sex offenders have not just wrecked their lives but have damaged the lives of others as well.

Most civilly committed sex offenders are keenly aware, at least, that they have wrecked their own lives. They are not where they want to be. They lack basic freedoms. They cannot go anywhere except the unit and the yard. The restrictions are similar to prison. They cannot shop or take a walk or drive a car until they are in the transitional program. There are myriad rules designed to keep order, to keep the units clean, to keep everyone safe. What they read and what they see are carefully controlled. I don't question these rules. I am well aware of the need for them. Still, it is hard to call the life of anyone committed as a sexually violent predator as successful in any way.

The psychopaths, of course, see it differently. They see the world through a lens of defiance and are always the heroes of their stories. Everyone is out for number one. They were just unlucky. They didn't commit offenses; they *caught charges*, like the rest of us catch colds. There are always people to prey on, especially in prison, so they never run out of entertainment. They believe they are unbroken and the rest of us are sheep. But this wears thin, even for them. Sometimes they enter what has been termed "the zero state," which seems

Chapter 16. Hope

more than anything like a state of boredom as much as it is a state of depression. Psychopaths need excitement to feel alive.

It is the others, however, the ones who know they have failed to build any kind of life worth having, that make me sad when I walk into a prison or a civil commitment center for sex offenders. Whether their behavior is the result of their genes, their upbringing, or their choices, these are wasted lives, lived without responsibility or concern for others, lives that have built nothing and destroyed much. And it is these offenders who have made me try to understand the role of hope and to conclude that hope is the holy grail of change.

In 2001, Shadd Maruna wrote a ground-breaking book on the difference in British criminals who continued to commit crimes versus those who stopped (persisters versus desisters or quitters). Of course, the first issue with a study of this type is the measurement of quitting crime. Maruna was dependent on self-report, not normally the most reliable of techniques with criminals. Still, there were definite differences in the two groups. One group had more cognitive distortions than the other, most notably an exaggerated and unrealistic belief in their control over their future. Surprisingly, it was the quitters who held the cognitive distortions, not the persisters. These cognitive distortions were usually unrealistic, and sometimes breathtakingly so.

> It was just that, um, I realized that the entire thing had all been an act, my entire life, all the criminal offenses, all me [sic] drug taking, it was all a sham.... It was just like what it was, was right at the core of me, I am who I am now, who I've always been inside. I've always been intelligent, right, inside. I've always been intelligent, honest, hard-working, truth, erm, nice, you know love ... it couldn't get out [Maruna, 2000, p. 92].

Whatever they had been in the past, it was definitely not hard-working and honest, but to those who quit offending they had *always* had these qualities. Their good qualities had heretofore been trapped, mostly due to outside forces, not their own choices. "The drink was killing me by the age of 21," one quitter said. "Heroin made me sneaky," said another. Even when they committed crimes, *they* didn't commit them. "*It* just happened to lapse." Their offenses were caused by something or someone else, and they were better than other offenders.

> I wasn't happy selling [drugs], you know. You're making money and whatever, it was just something that, what it was, it was the people that I'd come into contact with, selling it. I just didn't like.... It took me into a world, a seedy world that I didn't like.... I mean the low-life scum bags, low intelligence, you know. I had nothing in common [Maruna, 2000, p. 91].

They had an inflated, narcissistic, and missionary sense of purpose. They did not consider their past shameful. They considered it a necessary prelude to their future calling, which has been called the "redemption narrative."

The redemption narrative tended to follow a similar script:

- They were always good souls.
- They were victims of circumstance.
- They got "accidentally" involved with crime.
- It was a product of their childhoods.
- Now with help from an outside force, they can now accomplish what they were "meant to do."
- Now they must "give something back."

This is one reason so many alcohol and drug offenders seek professions as drug counselors. It justifies their entire history. Sometimes offenders even saw themselves as superior to the straight world:

> I believe that all recovering addicts are the Chosen Ones. That's my point of view. I feel we are all chosen by God, because we're loved.... The people who are not addicts, they're not—they still have their problems. People who are in recovery.... They learn how to live life on life's terms [Maruna, 2000, pp. 98–99].

Up until this study, the standard treatment for offenders, including sex offenders, was to insist they take responsibility for their

Chapter 16. Hope

offenses. But Maruna found that taking responsibility didn't distinguish the groups. It was hope that pulled them, not shame that drove them. While this must be integrated into treatment, there is still a case to be made for asking offenders, particularly sex offenders, to take responsibility for their offenses. If a sex offender does not admit and take responsibility for entering that house at 3 a.m., he won't examine the faulty thinking, poor decision-making, and cognitive distortions that got him there. And too, one could argue that the property offenders in this study differ in important ways from sex and violent offenders.

Still, there is no literature that supports shame as a therapeutic technique. Shame does not seem to be helpful in any way. Shame paralyzes. It creates resentment and a sense of utter failure. It doesn't move offenders anywhere except toward an attitude of "What the hell. It's too late now."

The fact that this grandiose and narcissistic rewriting of their personal histories could help to prevent future offending can be attributed to the sense of self-respect it gives them, to the sense of identity as a non-offending person it affords, and to the sense of hope it fosters.

The difficulty for therapists of sex and violent offenders is how to inspire hope without colluding with the various negative thinking errors that offenders have: what they did was not so bad, they are not as deviant as everybody else in the program, they won't do it again so they really don't need treatment, etc. Good therapists walk a knife edge, treating everyone with respect for their human potential while not minimizing the harmfulness of what they have done or their potential for future harm. Many therapists fall off this knife edge, either becoming angry and demeaning toward the offenders they work with or colluding and minimizing their behavior. The best therapists are capable of liking someone without trusting them, but that is hard for most people, whether they are therapists or not. It is the ability to separate likeability from trustworthiness that divides the effective change agent from the easily conned and colluding one, not the type of technique employed.

Most of us have lives where hope is taken for granted, and we do not have any idea what it is like to feel hopeless. Therapists who have worked with depressed patients know. Hopelessness sucks the life out of the depressed and correlates with suicide. "Hope is a good thing," Stephen King wrote, "maybe the best of things and no good thing ever dies" (King, 1982). Hope may well be the best of things, but it can die, and that is definitely not a good thing. I have read of men in homeless shelters who simply turn their faces to the wall and don't get out of bed unless they are driven out. That is where hopelessness leads.

When my son died, a friend brought over a cartoon. While this may seem the most offensive thing he could possibly have done, it actually resonated. The cartoon showed the feet of someone walking and the caption was along the lines of "Now if nothing bad happens and the earth keeps orbiting the sun it is possible my right foot may come into view at any moment." And that was how I felt. I could not look ahead more than the next few seconds. I could not count on anything. Life ceased being a gift and became a sentence. It was only when I had the possibility of having the other children I had always wanted that I developed hope and the ability to see a future that was not a form of torture.

For me, the hope I developed came not from rational thought but from a deep hunger that I only partially understood. Yes, I had wanted more children before my son died, but not with the kind of hunger that came afterward. I have often wondered if other parents who lost children had the hunger for more children run over them like a freight train as I did.

Hope matters not just to inmates or patients but to all of us, children most of all. Parents who tell their children they will never amount to anything are soul-killers. Once I was having lunch with friends, and the man, who was consistently down on his son for very little reason, asked me if I could take his son through a "scared straight program." I said I could not and would not if I could. I did not say what I thought but have regretted not doing so ever since. Had I been honest with him I'd have said:

Chapter 16. Hope

> You want to take your son to a prison and tell him he could end up there. You do that. The next time I'm in Cambridge, I'll take my kids to Harvard and tell them they could end up there.

For me, inspiring hope is a moral imperative because I am committed to therapeutic change and the decent treatment of human beings, regardless of their offenses. What little research we have on the subject indicates that telling yourself you will always be a failure is a self-fulling prophecy. You must have hope you can do better, to do better. Hope both precedes and follows change. But the hope that people are capable of doing better and the reality of whether they *are* doing better or faking it or even fooling themselves are different things. Hope does not replace the long, slow work of treatment, but it does motivate it.

Chapter 17

On the Problem with Power

I interviewed sex offenders for a decade in a nearby state to determine whether or not they met the criteria for civil commitment as sexually violent predators. After 10 years I obtained a contract to do evaluations in the same state to help determine who got out of the same civil commitment center. By law all sex offenders got a new evaluation each year to determine if they were ready for release. Some were people that I helped put in civil commitment, and I began seeing the effects of treatment, or the refusal of treatment, or the failure of treatment years down the line.

The job weighed on me. I found that when I said an offender was fit for release, I lived in fear he would reoffend. When I said he wasn't ready for release, I felt zero satisfaction in sending him back to a secure ward to waste his life, although I had no doubts that it was sometimes necessary. There are men and women who are simply too dangerous to be on the streets. For me, this kind of power implied a terrifying amount of responsibility with way too much at stake. It was oppressive. Of course, I only had a degree of power. Others were involved in making these decisions: therapists, attorneys, judges, and juries. But I had some say in these decisions, quite a bit if I did my job right, and I had no sense of ease with it. There is no scientific litmus test for who will reoffend and who won't, and the best we can do are probabilities—is he more likely or not to reoffend—and those were based on imperfect psychological tests. Having any degree of power over whether someone spends their life locked up was enough to keep me up at night. I am aware that some

Chapter 17. On the Problem with Power

spend their lives looking to have power over others, but I don't understand it.

"Maybe that makes you exactly the right person for the job," a friend said. "Would you really want someone in that position who enjoyed having power over others?"

It's a point. Anyone with any degree of power over others ought to feel uncomfortable, ought to feel burdened by it, ought to feel unsure. If so, they had the right woman for the job. Many years ago, David McClelland developed a theory that people were achievement oriented, affiliation oriented, and/or power oriented. Of course, almost everyone is a combination of the three, but the ratios differ from person to person. Affiliation orientation—yes, I understand that. I have children whose slightest up or down changes my heart rate and friends to whom I am intensely loyal. Achievement orientation—I won't even try to plea bargain. Guilty as charged. But power? Certainly, I have met people who enjoy having power over others—but why? When you have power over others, you are not just connected to them, you are to some degree *responsible* for them. It makes me shudder.

I live alone, except for my cats and dogs. The dog and I are buddies, and nobody has any power over cats. I am in private practice, so I don't have a boss or subordinates. When I need help, I contract with assistants who are enterprising and need no supervision. I can't even tolerate houseguests unless they are the sort that entertain themselves and feel free to hit the fridge when they are hungry between meals. I don't have a single friend who would have flunked the Milgram experiment. One of my closest women friends spent 10 years wandering from country to country picking up small jobs along the way. Freud would no doubt have a field day with me, and I can spell "counter-dependent," but at this point does it really matter why the cards fell this way? They're on the table. The point is, given how I am, I'm not necessarily in the best position to understand those who are either unnecessarily dependent on others or want to have power over them.

I don't deal a lot with dependence, but Lord, the power hungry are with us—those who manage to stay on the legal side of things and those who disregard the law entirely. I see the politicians and the executives on television, but I have little contact with them. They are rarely put in jail, and when they are, like Cosby—who was as dangerous as any offender I deal with—they often get out early because they can hire the lawyers to find the legal technicalities or for "good behavior." Most of my contacts are with those for whom prison is seen as an inevitable stop in their career path and who have often been in jail for other types of crimes as well.

If there are those who assault others because it is an easy way to make money, or rape them because it is easier and quicker than a hook-up, there are still others for whom the money and the rape are a means to an end. The high is the moment of defeat in the victim's eyes. The particular man I am interviewing today is an emotional sadist, someone for whom the betrayal is everything. A prison guard first met him when he was in his early 20s and looked 15. The guard took a liking to this "troubled" young man and wanted to help him. The guard and his family were religious, and the guard persuaded the young man to join a prison Bible study group. Before long, the guard's wife was also visiting. When the young man got out of prison, the officer and his wife agreed to let him live with them, even though he was a child molester and they had a nine-year-old daughter. He didn't have a valid driver's license, but he needed to drive to have a job, so the officer let him use his car to get back and forth. So now we have a correctional officer aiding and abetting a clear violation of the law and of the offender's parole. Of course, you can see where this is going. The offender molested the guard's daughter. At the time the molestations were going on, the guard and his wife were in the process of trying to adopt the offender.

When I interviewed the offender, he told me this:

> What helps me so much is I have something about me I can really attract people to me.... The person gets to really care and trust me. The problem I always had is where the excitement would come in. I would get them

Chapter 17. On the Problem with Power

to trust me, and I would set them up for the fall. It's almost like a power that you have. It's like a rush that you get from it.

Needless to say, his eyes lit up when he said this. He went on gushing:

It's like a rush. I really don't know how to explain it. I've never been into drugs real strong. From just what I have seen it's like somebody who's addicted to heroin or cocaine. An incredible feeling. Strongest at the end when I know I'm going to let them down in some way.

Of course, this isn't his first rodeo. He gave me other examples where he had developed the power to hurt someone by befriending them first. One was a young teen prostitute. Teen prostitutes have almost always been sexually abused, usually by a family member. Typically, they have run away from home and end up prostituting themselves in order to eat. He was well aware of her traumatized past and befriended her, making her feel better about herself and establishing himself as a safe refuge. This was all the set-up to the thrill. The thrill was the day he turned on her and said every hurtful thing his ingenious mind could come up with to tear her down.

Getting the person to trust me first. Then I knew I could do whatever I wanted. I wanted to see the pain I could cause them, the bringing them down. It was the ultimate rush.

In the case of the officer and his wife, the denouement came when they found out he was sexually abusing their daughter.

The best part I just basically told them you are so fucking stupid. You know I am a sex offender. I have child victims. You are stupid enough. You and your wife both. You are fucking morons. Everything that's happened to you—you deserve.

Given how much he enjoyed power and control, and hurting people, I asked him if he had ever been physically sadistic. He replied:

I've never been physical.... Kind of what I felt is when you hurt someone physically, that goes away. When you hurt someone emotionally, that never goes away. That was the thrill.

He was arrested and returned to prison. Rumor has it a probation officer was fired for letting him live with the guard's family. But—almost unbelievably—the officer and his wife kept trying to visit the offender. They wanted to understand how he could do such a thing. They believed—they still wanted to believe—that everyone can be redeemed, that people are basically good, that love and kindness will fix anything. The offender said to his therapist, "I feel like saying, 'What the fuck is wrong with you, lady? I molested your fucking daughter.'" Fortunately, he was moved to a treatment program that denied the visits. That is a good thing because I believe fervently, had the offender not tired of the game, had he produced enough tears and enough show of remorse, he could have done the same thing all over again.

I was working on a film about staff manipulation at the time, and this man agreed to participate. I knew from the moment that he agreed that he was likely setting me up. I just didn't know when the denouement would come. I thought it would possibly happen immediately after the filming so I told the cameramen if the offender said he had changed his mind and was withdrawing his consent, they should calmly pack up as though they had a million other offenders to film and his refusal was of no consequence or interest to them. He could withdraw permission if he chose, but I would not give him the satisfaction of seeing the disappointment that he craved.

He waited. It was a week later that I got a message from the social worker that he wanted to talk to me. He said he was afraid that the film might somehow end up in court and he was thinking about withdrawing his permission to use it. I was supposed to come back to the prison and talk to him about it. Had I done so, he would have vacillated back and forth, drawing the visits out as long as possible and then he would have finally said no, only when I was there in person, of course. I told the social worker I wasn't coming back. He could withdraw from the project if he chose by writing me, but if he thought that would stop a judge from subpoenaing the footage, he was mistaken. I would comply with any subpoena that came. Of

Chapter 17. On the Problem with Power

course, one never came because he withdrew permission, so the film never saw the light of day.

That wasn't the point anyway. The point was to do to me what he had done to others. I was supposed to be so taken with the rapport between us, with how candidly he described his past exploits that I thought I was special, different, that I had a connection with him that others didn't. I was supposed to get excited about the film and then be deflated and hurt when he finally pulled the plug—after he toyed with me for a while.

It is a mistake to think how people treat others is different from how they will treat us, that somehow we are different and special. I have a friend who was getting married to a woman who had previously been married five times and had walked out on each marriage after two years without explanation. "But they were all jerks," he told me. I said, "You do know what's going to happen, right?" But love is deaf. And guess what happened two years later.

The difficulty is that humans trust because we need each other. Humans are not lone tigers patrolling their territory. It is our ability to cooperate with each other that won the day against the ice, the tiger, and the bear—not our impressive claws or fast running speed. But sheep who can't recognize a wolf in sheepskin are vulnerable. Asking people to be discriminating in trusting others and to rely on actions more than words turns out to be a hill too high for some adults and all children to climb. It also means that those who betray trust strike at the heart of our mammalian needs, and there are victims who do not recover. They no longer believe they know who to trust and thus trust no one. This is a terrifying way to live. I grit my teeth when people claim that the incestuous father, the Cosby-type groomer, the family infiltrator are less dangerous because they don't use overt violence (at least in Cosby's case, when people were conscious). They are not looking at the impact on the victim of losing the capacity to trust and no longer being able to believe in their own judgment. Betrayal trauma, as Jennifer Freyd and colleagues have shown, is real and as dangerous as being hit by a two-by-four in the head.

The belief that we are different, and he won't do to us or to our children what he has done to others, is to engage in misplaced hope, projection, denial, or even narcissism. How people treat others has to do with who they are, not who their targets are. Too much trust and you will find yourself hearing siren calls from the rocks as Odysseus did. Listen to them at your peril. In the case of the emotional sadist above, the comparison is more than apt. The lure of the sirens' songs was that they promised Odysseus knowledge, and I was seeking knowledge of this offender's methods and techniques.

Like Odysseus, I was trying to learn something but had no desire to end up on the rocks. He had to tie himself to the mast to keep from being lured to his destruction. Of course, Odysseus didn't have the advantage that the sirens had sat down with him ahead of time and explained exactly how they went about their business as I did.

People who aren't wired to exploit others, and who don't have a strong power orientation, too often see the world as though such motivations don't exist. This offender's make-up was beyond the officer and his wife's reach or understanding. They were deeply religious and saw the world through a philosophy which told them that there is good in everyone and that everyone can be redeemed: all prodigal sons can come home. But I can hear the reader scoff. It's obvious something was wrong with the officer and his wife, you say. I would disagree. The officer and his wife were only taking their religion seriously, so much so that they could not see the bad in this man, only the hope that he was serious about turning a new leaf.

Religion revolves around the concept of evil; certainly, psychology has been slow to embrace it. Much of psychological theory is geared toward explaining (and sometimes excusing) behaviors that others consider evil. And yet offenders will tell you that religious people are the easiest to con. "They try to see the good in everyone," as one offender said. No wonder religion put the devil in hell, which—like heaven—is over there somewhere. Here on Earth, everyone can be redeemed.

Chapter 17. On the Problem with Power

These beliefs do not always serve religious folk well. Seeing good in everyone is a wonderful sentiment but an impractical way to live your life. This isn't heaven, folks. Eve would have been better off had she eyed the serpent a little more skeptically and wondered about his motivations.

Chapter 18

The Conman and the Courts

On Sunday, May 25, 2003, I flew to Kentucky for a court case, but the opposing expert never showed up. On Monday the court was informed that the expert, Richard Gardner, had killed himself that weekend, and the case was postponed. As 20 years have now passed, I can no longer remember the details of the case, but I remember distinctly the reason I went. It was the first opportunity I had to go up directly against Gardner, a man who had developed a theory that held 90 percent of disclosures of paternal sexual abuse by children whose parents were divorcing was a lie, coached or enabled by the mother. He paid lip service to the idea that 10 percent might be accurate, but he never seemed to find a case where he believed it was. Even if there was no evidence of coaching, he thought that if the mother believed the child's disclosure, she should be subject to sanctions, up to and including losing custody. Custody should instead be given to the accused father. Gardner described what the mother should do if her child disclosed sexual abuse during or after a divorce in the documentary *Small Justice: Little Justice in America's Family Courts*. Mothers were told to say to their child, "I don't believe you. I'm going to beat you for saying it. Don't ever talk that way again about your father."

The bar should be high when taking a child from their mother, but one will look in vain for *any* scientific evidence to support this theory. There is none. The lack of scientific evidence never bothered Gardner. Gardner was not a researcher and once developed a scale called the Indices of Pedophilia for determining if a man was

Chapter 18. The Conman and the Courts

a pedophile—which he never tested for validity or reliability but nonetheless introduced as a way to determine if a man was guilty of child molestation. He did not mention there was a difference in child molesters and pedophiles. Pedophiles have a sexual preference for children, but the term child molester simply denotes that the individual has molested a child. Offenders do so for a variety of reasons; many are not pedophiles. Most incest offenders, particularly, do not have a sexual preference for children and would not be classified as pedophiles. Most of the items on Gardner's scale didn't even correlate with child molestation or pedophilia and included the following:

- low intellectual level;
- psychosis;
- coercive-dominating behavior;
- passivity and impaired self-assertion (the opposite of the previous item);
- large collection of child pornography;
- career choice that brings him into contact with children;
- use of rationalizations that support child molestation;
- lack of cooperation in the evaluation;
- childhood history of child sexual abuse; and
- unconvincing denial.

Think of some of the famous child molesters out there: Michael Jackson, Roman Polanski, Woody Allen, Jerry Sandusky, for example. Do any of those offenders strike you as lacking in intelligence, as being psychotic, or as even being known for having a large collection of child pornography? Just those 10 items alone offered protection to any offender who was of normal intelligence, not psychotic, and denied he was abused as a child. If he was on his best behavior in front of a custody evaluator (the child's account and the mother's were worthless in Gardner's system) and had not been found with a large collection of child pornography, he earned more points on the Gardner scale. Offenders who did not work with children and were willing to be interviewed continued to rack up points. If he was smooth in his denial—and many offenders, as we have seen in previous chapters, are very persuasive—he was granted even more points.

Most incest offenders, and even most extrafamilial pedophiles, would pass this test. Pretty much everything was wrong with Gardner's scale, and it was never accepted in the field of psychology, which has strict standards for the development of psychological tests. Not surprisingly, such tests have to demonstrate that they can reliably detect what their authors claim they can detect.

But Gardner had more success with his invention of the "parental alienation syndrome" (PAS) which he developed in the '80s. He made that up too, and it also lacked empirical backing—and still does—but it answered a need and became an easy answer when children disclosed child sexual abuse in the middle of divorce cases or even after a divorce. Judges didn't have to take the word of a seven-year-old over that of an educated, articulate adult male with status in the community. They didn't have to brand the child a liar either. The problem, the theory claimed, was not the innocent child, it was the mother, and mothers have been beat up by psychology before. Whether it was the claim that "cold fish" mothers caused autism, the allegation that women were hysterical and imagined sexual offenses against them, or the theory that incest was a case of mothers acting out their homosexual desires through the "vehicle" father, psychology has a poor track record when it comes to misogyny (Salter, 1988).

Gardner's original formulation stated that

> the Parental Alienation Syndrome (PAS) is a disorder that arises primarily in the context of child-custody disputes.... The disorder's primary manifestation is the child's campaign of denigration against a parent, a campaign that has no justification because the target parent has always been a good, loving parent. The disorder results from the combination of a programming (brainwashing) parent's indoctrinations and the child's own contributions to the vilification of the target parent. When true parental abuse and/or neglect is present, the child's animosity may

Chapter 18. The Conman and the Courts

be justified, and so the parental alienation syndrome explanation for the child's alienation is not applicable [Gardner, 2002].

Gardner's observations that children are sometimes estranged from one parent and align with the other in divorce cases are true. Children sometimes do pick sides and reject the other parent. However, his claim that alienation in custody cases routinely results from brainwashing by the mother (Gardner, 1992) has no evidence to support it (Bruch, 2001; Clemente & Padilla-Racero, 2016; Faller, 1998; Hoult, 2006). The causes of refusal of parental contact are varied. Wallerstein and Kelly's 25-year study of children of divorcing parents found that children between the ages of 9 and 12 often rejected one parent and aligned with the other, generally rejecting the parent they blamed for the divorce (Wallerstein & Kelly, 1980; Wallerstein et al., 2001) It was a phase, though, and every child in their study who did so reconciled with the rejected parent, often within a year or two and all before the age of 18. Huff's study of 292 young adults who were children of divorce and rejected contact with one parent found that children aligned with the parent who exhibited the most warmth toward them (Huff, 2015).

While some causes of a child refusing contact are developmental, abuse and neglect can also cause parental rejection (Huff, 2015). A sexually abusing father is likely to have an estranged child who doesn't want to see him and sides with the mother in a divorce. Rejection based on abuse is unlikely to resolve so quickly. Likewise, a child who has been beaten or neglected or whose mother has been beaten may also reject the abuser. Before it can be claimed that the problem is one parent implanting unfounded ideas into a child's brain, developmental processes must be ruled out, as must the possibility of abuse, especially when the child is the one reporting abuse. Gardner paid lip service to the concept that parental rejection could be based on abuse in his definition, but it was only lip service: as noted, he claimed that 90 percent of disclosures of abuse in custody cases were the result of PAS (Gardner, 1987, p. 67).

Gardner developed a test he called the Sexual Abuse Legitimacy Scale (SALS) to determine if the disclosed abuse was genuine or fabricated. This scale had no psychometric properties; neither reliability nor validity was ever established. In short, there was no evidence that it would do what he claimed it could do, separating out true and false cases of sexual abuse.

One of the items on the SALS was whether the disclosure occurred in the middle of a custody evaluation. Thus, a scale that was supposed to determine whether the abuse had occurred in child custody cases had an item that said if the disclosure occurred in the middle of a custody case, it was a false report. Catch-22, anyone? Gardner was forced to withdraw this scale, just like his previous one on offenders, as it too had no scientific basis.

Gardner admitted that he set the cut-off points on this scale to favor the accused fathers, saying, "I have chosen to recommend a cutoff point that *might* indeed exonerate bona fide perpetrators in order to protect innocents [fathers] who might be falsely considered guilty" (Gardner, 1987, p. 186). Given Gardner's recommendation that custody be transferred from the mother to the father in cases where PAS was found, he made a clear choice to transfer children to some offenders rather than take the chance that an "innocent" man might not gain custody. He justified this by saying he stood by the "American legal principle that 'it is better to let 100 men go free than convict one innocent man'" (Gardner, 1987, p. 174). However, the American legal principle said nothing about handing over children to likely abusers in non-criminal cases based on artificially engineered cut-off points, derived from an unproven test with items that has never been shown to distinguish truth cases from false ones.

He does not appear to have thought that badly of pedophilia in any case. He wrote, "It is extremely important that the evaluator appreciate that sexual activities between an adult and a child are *an ancient tradition* and have been found to exist to a significant degree in just about every society in history that has been studied in depth" (Gardner, 1992, p. 46; italics mine). He wrote:

Chapter 18. The Conman and the Courts

> Women and children, being weaker than men, have been easily exploited by the more powerful. However, and this is an extremely important point, such encounters are *not* necessarily traumatic. The determinant as to whether the experience will be traumatic is the social attitude towards these encounters. As Hamlet said: There is nothing either good or bad, but thinking makes it so [Gardner, 1992, p. 670].

Apparently, if society approved of women and children being exploited by men, such exploitation was not traumatic. One wonders if he thought the same of slavery. Gardner argued that pedophilia was beneficial to the species in that it increased a child's sexualization and thus every form of human sexual conduct was positive because it increased the likelihood of reproduction (Gardner, 1992, p. 24). He thought all paraphilias—including sadism, rape, necrophilia, bestiality, pedophilia, and coprophilia (sexual interest in feces)—served the purposes of the species by increasing sexual excitation (Gardner 1992, p. 20).

He argued that there was no good definition of pedophilia and wrote, "My final position on this matter is this: a *pedophile* is the name given to a person whom the judge and/or jury decides they want to put away" (Gardner, 1992, p. 46). Even when abuse was proven he thought that therapists would "do well to be very cautious about bringing about a situation in which they promulgate alienation of a child from a parent, even the parent who has sexually abused the child" (Gardner, 1992, p. 537). Offenders, he thought, might well stop the abuse just because of the exposure, even if they were exonerated.

It is extremely odd that he took the risk to children and the trauma inflicted on them by sexual abuse so lightly and was so very supportive of pedophiles. It is also ironic that he thought therapists should avoid a situation where they "promulgate alienation" from an abuser, but he routinely recommended separation from the mother and full custody to fathers in cases of "parental alienation syndrome." He took no account of whether the mother was the child's major attachment figure.

Gardner went so far as to state that a mother who was neutral about visitation and said it was up to the child if she or he wanted to visit the father was a sign of a fabricated report because the mother was implicitly communicating criticism of the father. Even the mother hiring an attorney or a mental health professional to see the child was considered by Gardner to be a sign of a fabricated report and were included in his screen (Gardner, 1987, p. 197). Any action she took to protect the child—asking for supervised visitation with the father, trying not to force a child to visit the other parent, taking the child for medical exams, taking the child to a therapist—were all evidence in Gardner's system that the mother was an "alienator," even though these are exactly the steps we would expect loving mothers to take if their child disclosed sexual abuse. Gardner has called the mothers' attorneys and therapists who supported the child "hired guns," but apparently considered the fathers' attorneys and expert witnesses to be fair-minded.

Items for the father included weak or unconvincing denial and the presence of other sexual deviations. If the father professed his innocence and no one knew of any other sexual deviations, this counted toward considering the disclosure a false report.

Although he had no science behind his claim, he wrote that in custody litigation "the vast majority of children who profess sexual abuse are fabricators" (Gardner, 1987, p. 274). Gardner simply made this up. There has *never* been any empirical support for this view. Indeed, research has found that few custody cases involve reports of sexual abuse (Thoennes & Tjaden, 1990), and some research has found that the rate of false reports in custody cases is no higher than in cases of child sexual abuse that did not involve custody issues (Brown et al., 1997; Schuman, 2000).

PAS has been interpreted and used by Gardner and his followers, who have renamed it parental alienation, to say that mental health professionals and courts should not listen to children who say they have been abused if the disclosures arise during a divorce, his initial description notwithstanding. Part of the evidence for Gardner's belief that such disclosures were fabricated was that the mothers

Chapter 18. The Conman and the Courts

were often angry at the fathers, but in fact, people on both sides of divorce cases are frequently angry. As one website on divorce stated, "The idea of the friendly divorce seems plausible to people who have never been divorced." But if she wasn't angry before the disclosure, the mother was definitely likely to be angry afterward. It would be unfair to say Gardner thought mothers shouldn't be angry following a disclosure of child sexual abuse by a father. He thought they should be angry—at the child.

If both mother and child believed the child had been abused, they had *folie á deux*, a shared delusion. If the child disclosed sexual abuse and both the child, the mother, *and* the therapist believed the child had been abused, they had a *folie á trois*. They were all psychotic. PAS has been used and *is still being used*, not as an explanation after other sources of alienation have been ruled out, but to invalidate children's disclosures of sexual abuse.

A theory that cannot be falsified is not a theory; it is a polemic. In Gardner's system, the fact that the child discloses at all is considered evidence of parental alienation. Although Gardner admitted that some men molest children in the middle of a divorce, there was no possible way for an abused child to tell Gardner or his followers that would be accepted. If a child told a therapist, he believed therapists should contradict the child when they tried to talk about it and say, "That didn't happen! So let's go and talk about *real* things, like your next visit with your father" (Gardner, 2000, p. 202). He noted that the therapist "must have a thick skin and be able to tolerate the shrieks and claims of impending maltreatment that PAS children often profess" (Gardner, 2000, p. 201).

He assured judges that recalcitrant children actually wanted to be forced to visit so they have an excuse to do so. "I cannot emphasize this point strongly enough. PAS children want to be forced" (Gardner, 2002, p. 9). He not only believed in arguing with children in therapy that they were not abused, but he also believed in putting children and the alleged abuser *together* in his office in the evaluation phase to "allow for a free flow of communication between the two parties and give the accused a much greater opportunity to prove his or her innocence" (Gardner, 1987, p. 141). Certainly, a meeting with a child's abuser would not likely give the child much chance to prove the offender's guilt. Gardner gave no weight at all to the power differential between parent and child, especially when the parent was abusive, nor did he even mention in passing assessing whether the child had PTSD or affective flashbacks about abuse that would make the visit traumatic. After all, the child was not abused. He could tell because the child disclosed in the middle of a divorce and the mother was angry at the father and supported the child.

Gardner willfully misunderstood children's desires in other ways, stating that a child who disclosed sexual abuse by a father was often hiding a desire to have sex with him. Children were dealing with their sexual impulses by claiming the opposite:

> Instead of saying, "I would love to have some sexual involvement with my father," she can say, "I hate having a sexual relationship with my father." Yet, the fantasy in both cases may be very similar if not identical ... the child is essentially saying, "It is not I who want him to rape me, it is he who wants to rape me." This too is guilt assuaging [Gardner, 1992, p. 537].

Gardner proposed that in "moderate cases" of PAS, child support should be reduced if the mother failed to religiously honor visitation. If that failed, the mother should be placed on house arrest for periods of time. If that failed, she should wear an ankle bracelet. If that still didn't work, she should be put in jail. This was for moderate cases. For more "severe" cases, the courts should remove the child from the custody of the mother if she believed the child's disclosures and did not encourage unsupervised visitation. The father should be given full custody, and the child restricted from seeing the mother at all for up to several weeks, to be replaced with restricted supervised visitation for the mother, which Gardner thought should be as little as two to four hours a week. He recommended a transitional deprogramming camp for the child to convince the child she had not been abused.

Chapter 18. The Conman and the Courts

Depriving a child suddenly of their major attachment figure is an astonishing recommendation. Psychology has an entire field of study devoted to issues of attachment in children, and there is consensus that attachment figures play a major role in the child's development. By definition, in the cases Gardner cited, the child was not attached to the father and was attached to the mother. To take a child from their major attachment figure and hand them off to a parent they were not attached to—no matter the reason—is to essentially put the child through a maternal death. Gardner didn't see it that way. He thought that removing the child from any father—regardless of abuse—would deal a devastating blow to the child's psychological development, but that the child would quickly recover from being pried from the mother, regardless of the degree of attachment.

Batterers and sexual abusers have both taken advantage of Gardner's theories and the willingness of the legal system to accept them. As Joan Meier, National Family Violence Law Center Professor of Clinical Law and Director of the National Family Violence Law Center at the George Washington University Law School, points out:

> It is well-established that an abuser's active undermining of his partner's authority and competence to parent is one of the most common and most destructive elements of the abusive relationship....
>
> Batterers' vendettas against their children's mothers are also often played out in aggressive litigation against her, especially over custody....
>
> Given the degree to which abusers utilize alienating behaviors to undermine mothers' relationships with their children, a Martian who had just landed on earth might ask why advocates for domestic violence victims are so hostile to the theory of parental alienation: Is it not exactly what batterers have been doing all these years, and is it not a bad thing? Yes, and yes, but that is not how alienation theory was derived, propounded, or implemented. Instead, alienation theory's traction in family courts is fueled by the denial of abuse; it is used to refute mothers' claims of paternal abuse and almost never to recognize the emotional abuse many abusers inflict on their children [Meier, 2009, pp. 233–234].

An entire series of research articles have been written by respected professionals in the field pointing out all these flaws in the theory and many more (Berg, 2011; Clemente & Padilla-Racero, 2016; Dallam & Silberg, 2016; Faller, 1998; Hoult, 2006; Meier, 2009; Meier & Dickson, 2017; Neilson, 2018; O'Donohue et al., 2016; Rüdiger, 2015). Jennifer Hoult's article is a particularly meticulous and thorough compendium of research related to the evidentiary admissibility and scientific validity of PAS. Generally circumspect voices have been driven to exasperation by Gardner's claims and have used terms rarely heard in academia. Carol Bruch quoted Paul Fink, past president of the American Psychological Association, as saying, "PAS as a scientific theory has been excoriated by legitimate researchers across the nation. Judged solely on his merits, Dr. Gardner should be a rather pathetic footnote or an example of poor scientific standards" (Bruch, 2001). Jon Conte, an icon in the field, was quoted as saying that the Sexual Abuse Legitimacy Scale was "probably the most unscientific piece of garbage I've seen in the field in all my time." An article by Thomas and Richardson was titled "30 Years On and Still Junk Science" (2015). Meier wrote:

> The dominant census in the scientific community is that there is *no scientific evidence of PAS*. PAS is a label that offers a particular *explanation* for a breach in relationship between a child and parent, but insofar as that breach could be explained in other ways, it is not in itself a medical or psychological diagnosis.... While clinicians frequently insist that they often see "alienation" in their caseloads (Johnston and Kelly 2004) there is no objective way to verify whether the relationship breaches they observe are caused by an alienation "disorder" as opposed to a "healthy response" to a destructive or disconnected parent.

The American Psychological Association refused to include parental alienation syndrome or parental alienation in *The Diagnostic and Statistical Manual of Mental Disorders, Fifth Edition* (DSM 5). The National Council of Juvenile and Family Court Judges issued a report stating:

> The theory positing the existence of "PAS" has been discredited by the scientific community.... Any testimony that a party to a custody case

Chapter 18. The Conman and the Courts

suffers from the syndrome or "parental alienation" should therefore by ruled inadmissible and/or stricken from the evaluation report under both the standards in *Daubert* and the earlier *Frye* standard [Dalton et al., 2006, p. 24].

But the experts have just been shouting into the wind. The lack of scientific validity has not even slowed down the Gardner train. His theory makes things simple. One judge spoke of the "jolt of truth" she felt when she first read Gardner's work. She thought he had "just handed me the key to the mysteries of all my high-conflict family law custody cases ... the magic of the theory was intoxicating" (Slabach, 2014). That particular judge came to think that parent/child alienation might not be the answer to *all* cases of parental rejection by a child and that parental rejection had a number of different causes, abuse among them. It is unclear how many cases she decided before she came to that realization. Many in the legal system have drunk the whole pitcher of Kool-Aid, unimpressed by the lack of scientific validity. An article in the *Pasadena Star News* in 2014 quoted family court presiding judge Aviva Bobb as saying that just because there was no scientific evidence "doesn't mean that it does not exist." It doesn't mean it does, either. I doubt that many people would have surgery based on a theory that lacked any scientific evidence to back it up.

I have moments where I want to climb on a soap box in Times Square and scream about this. It is frustrating beyond belief to see such biased and shoddy work and have court after court give it credence. The cost to children who dare to disclose abuse once the offender is out of the house is incalculable. When I sent this book to an editor for review, she said the theory sounded insane and wanted to know what era it was popular in. This era. Parental alienation is popular to this day in a multitude of U.S. courts. People believe what they choose to believe and this can mean disregarding a wide chorus of professionals who are appalled by the acceptance of this theory.

The fact that it targets mothers may well be a factor in its success. Meier did a study of 238 published online opinions in battering or child sexual or child physical abuse custody cases between 2002 and 2013 (Meier & Dickson, 2017). She found that fathers who *merely alleged* alienation won their cases 2.3 times more than the mothers did. Child sexual abuse *allegations* actually increased the father's chances of winning. She also found that when the alienation was credited, the differences were even more pronounced. In seven cases, the courts found the father abusive and the mother alienating. The father won custody in all seven cases. Alienation trumped abuse, even though abuse in itself alienates children.

I once attended a Gardner training hoping to find what evidence he had to make such sweeping claims. I did not find any evidence and was astonished to find that the humor he used was almost entirely scatological. I left early. I can tolerate discussions of poop from a four-year-old, but they wear thin when told by an adult who is telling them instead of citing evidence to support a theory that is routinely used to discredit children's disclosures of sexual abuse.

I regret missing my chance to debate Gardner in court because of his untimely death. A document purporting to be the complete autopsy report by Laura S. Carbone, M.D., of Bergen County, New Jersey, has appeared online in multiple places, and it states that he had four stab wounds in his chest, one of which penetrated his heart and aorta. There were five wounds to his neck, most of which were superficial but one of which transected the right jugular vein. There were two superficial lacerations on the top and left of his forehead. The medical examiner declared his death a suicide, based apparently on his son's statement that Gardner had been distraught over the advancing symptoms of reflex sympathetic dystrophy, a painful neurological syndrome. Still, if it was suicide, it was an exceedingly odd one. Dr. Gardner had hydrocodone and fentanyl in his system, both backing up his son's claims that he had an intractable and excruciatingly painful medical condition, but also suggesting he had far easier ways to die than by stabbing himself to death. Cuts across the forehead seem particularly unusual for a suicide as forehead cuts would be very unlikely to result in death.

Chapter 18. The Conman and the Courts

I doubt my testimony against Gardner's theory would have done any good. It is such an *intoxicating* theory, and it makes things so simple. Children weren't really being abused. It was all the fault of the mothers.

Long ago, we reached the limits of my vision. I do not understand this hostility toward children who disclose sexual abuse and the enmity toward their mothers. In previous books, I have tracked it through the last hundred years of psychology, but I remain ignorant of its fundamental causes. Over 40 years ago, the legendary social worker and writer Florence Rush railed against what she called "this relentless tendency to blame women for male sexual transgression" (Rush, 1980, p. 194). Forty years ago. Why is it so hard to believe that men molest children, and why is it never their fault when they do?

Chapter 19

Society and Sex Offenders

Usually, I am a rational person who can discuss virtually anything with some detachment. Virtually anything. Crooked, lying politicians are an exception and so is the naïve way society, in general, and juries, experts and therapists, in particular, view sex offenders. It's the paradox in society's treatment of sex offenders that causes me to foam at the mouth. Sex offenders that the individual doesn't know personally are monsters, but sex offenders in the individual's family, among their acquaintances, or even within their community are not sex offenders at all, but innocent men being framed by someone: therapists, children, or mothers.

Recently I was asked to read and endorse a book on sex offenders an esteemed colleague and friend was publishing. I like this man. He is brilliant and kind and does impeccable research. But the book began by comparing sex offenders to victims of racial discrimination and witches burned at the stake. Moral panic was the theme, the notion that society over-estimates and over-reacts to some forms of risk, currently the risk that sex offenders will reoffend.

I don't disagree with everything my colleague says. Currently we have ill-advised and poorly-researched laws on sex offenders that often do more harm than good. If my colleague had merely said that, then he and I would be nodding in agreement. For example, for those who think residency restrictions will decrease sexual offending, I have one word: cars. Sex offenders typically get their victims through their vocation or avocation, rather than through geographic distribution. They are teachers and pediatricians and ministers and

Chapter 19. Society and Sex Offenders

tutors. They run youth choirs and Little League teams and teach music. They all drive cars. They don't usually find their victims in their neighborhoods. Some are parents, siblings, grandparents, and cousins who get their victims through their family relationships.

Of course, the vast majority of the people in professions that deal with children are legitimate, but if you are a pedophile who wants to find children, then you will be looking for a career or hobby that puts you in direct contact with them. Unsupervised contact. Trusted contact. Preferably overnight contact. Contact that gives you regular access and time to build a relationship. Even as I write this, I am embroiled in a case against a major youth organization. Youth-serving organizations fight an incessant battle trying to identify and combat sexual offenders who have infiltrated their ranks. Even when they do their job well, they are at risk. When they do it badly, they are fodder for camouflaged predators. In this case the organization did not even talk to a child after he had called up his mother on a camping trip with the offender and begged to come home. The offender refused to take him, even with the mother's request, and the police had to show up at the campsite to get him to take the boy home. Nonetheless, the organization accepted the offender's claim that the mother was overprotective and the boy a whiner and never even spoke to the boy. They just gave the offender another boy to mentor, who was, not surprisingly, also sexually abused and whose parents sued.

Residency requirements do nothing to prohibit contact through the main ways that offenders access children. There is research on this, and it agrees with what common sense would tell us: residency restrictions do not reduce sexual offending. Unfortunately, sometimes, instead, they put offenders further away from needed services that might reduce offending. As far as the sex offender registry is concerned, I think people ought to think long and hard before they put a 15-year-old who has committed one sexual offense on it. Of course, there are exceptions: an offense as serious as the rape and torture of a toddler, for instance, would warrant registration as opposed to a 15-year-old with a 13-year-old girlfriend.

But the paradox is that while the public is ready and willing to damn sex offenders in the abstract, the issue changes when they know one or even hear him testify. Sex offenders are "creeps," they say, and my child's teacher is a nice man, so it must be a false report. Or I saw that mom with her child, and she didn't seem like a sex offender to me. Or that man tenderly wiped his infant's nose in my office. He couldn't have physically abused her.[1] Or this man on the stand has done everything the treatment program has asked of him, and they still won't let him go. He deserves a chance. But there were reasons they didn't want to let him go.

Most sex offenders don't reoffend, the book I am reviewing says, but the reality is we really don't know that much about re-offense rates. We only know about getting-caught rates, and a large body of research tells us sex offenders commit far more offenses than they are caught for. A series of epidemiological studies have shown that only somewhere between 12 and 16 percent of child molestations ever come to the attention of authorities while the victims are children (see, for example, London, 2005). (Of course, a report when they are an adult is generally barred by the statute of limitations.) These data are based on surveys of adult survivors who were asked whether and to whom they disclosed their sexual abuse as children. Two-thirds never told anyone and the third that did often swore that person to secrecy. It bears repeating. Recidivism rates are not re-offense rates; they are getting-caught rates, rates of charges and convictions. Even most of the abused children who did tell someone did not tell someone who called the police. An offender I evaluated was typical. He was caught for six rapes, but admitted he committed 20. And he's a rapist. Rapists tend to have lower numbers of victims than child molesters, who have often committed hundreds of undetected offenses. But the opposing expert witness used generic getting-caught rates to argue he was unlikely to reoffend. Of course, he could have and would have said that each of the previous 19 times the man did reoffend.

Chapter 19. Society and Sex Offenders

Under water, there are certainly predatory sharks, but every fish from a minnow to a tuna recognizes them and stays away. Of course, sharks don't make much attempt at concealment. There are octopi who can do an amazingly accurate imitation of almost anything, including seaweed or rocks. God knows how many I have swam by unknowingly.[2] But I have met people and seen juries to whom you could show a video of the octopus changing into an exact replica of waving seaweed that would say, "Well, maybe he used to be an octopus, but that looks like seaweed now." Slow the film down. Show it again and again. It's the same critter. See him pretend he is seaweed. Now see him change back into an octopus and swim away. Admire his capacity for concealment, if you will, but understand who he is. "Nope, looks like seaweed to me." It is not the offenders I cannot contend with. It is the naïve people who enable them.

Before I wrote this chapter, I testified in the annual review of a sexually violent predator case. The man involved was the one described above as being caught for six rapes but having 20. He was committed as a sexually violent predator three and a half years ago. He had rocketed through the program, doing his homework meticulously, attending groups, and saying the right things. He had two therapists in that period of time and neither they nor I bought it that he had reformed. For one thing, he had a history of faking his way through treatment in the past and then reoffending afterward. For another thing, his offenses were gratuitously violent and that was the one thing he wouldn't admit.

He had arrests for six rapes. Some got dismissed as part of plea bargains, but he admitted under threat of a polygraph that he committed all of them plus 14 others. This is not surprising to people in my field. Research has found that sex offenders commit many more offenses than they are caught for and will admit it, sometimes, if you even tell them they will have to take a polygraph afterward. But say what you will about rapists—they differ in their degree of violence. Whereas many rapists threaten to kill their victims or even pull a knife or gun, they do not all put victims in the hospital. But he was on the extreme violence side of things. A sample of his rapes: he saw a woman he knew at a bar and talked her into going out to his car with him to smoke some marijuana. The woman was a thalidomide baby. Her mother had taken thalidomide when she was in utero, and as a result, she had a deformed arm that was more like a flipper and a deformed vagina that could not sustain intercourse. She was less than five feet tall and weighed less than 80 pounds. He attacked her in the car and started choking her. She couldn't breathe and scratched him. He beat her head on the car windows, hit her in the face multiple times, tried to tear off her deformed arm, and continued to strangle her. She agreed to have oral sex with him to save her life but told him her vagina was deformed and she couldn't have intercourse. He nonetheless tried to force his penis in her vagina. When it was finally over and he left her, she was bleeding from every orifice. Another example: he raped another woman in front of her three-year-old son, strangling her unconscious. Strangling was not unusual for him. It was his main method of not only subduing victims but also of maintaining his arousal. Another victim stated he put his penis inside her and then started strangling her. He was not strangling her to subdue her as he had already overpowered her. He was strangling her because it was exciting for him.

    He took the stand and in a meek and calm voice admitted his offenses. But he did not admit that he was sexually aroused by violence, and he lied about knowing the woman's vagina was deformed. He was only looking for love and acceptance, he told the jury, and he thought that's what sex meant.

    I took the stand also, and I testified to his entire violent past. I showed places in the records where he had admitted the victim told him her vagina was deformed. I told the jury that he was a smart man, and it was not credible to say that he thought if a woman was strangled into submission, she was loving and accepting him. This seemed obvious to me, and I thought it had to be obvious to the jury.

    His current therapist took the stand and stated he was not ready even for a transitional release program, much less outright

Chapter 19. Society and Sex Offenders

discharge. But she had to admit he had high marks in treatment. She had told me privately that whenever she had to score his treatment progress, she got physically sick. The way the items were framed, she had no choice but to give him high marks. For example, one item read, "he gives constructive feedback to others in 75% of his groups." A psychopath is always ready to give advice to others and can be quite insightful. Not surprisingly with his callousness and his track record, he had a high score on psychopathy. He had no conscience but could mimic one in a New York minute.

I left after my testimony, confident that this offender, one of the two or three worst offenders in the entire civil commitment program, would not be put in a transitional release program. I was right about that. I got the call a couple of days later when the trial was over. The jury outright discharged him to the community. He was a free man.

I have a habit of not knowing when to quit. I played basketball in pick-up games against men for decades until the day my back spasmed so badly I had to crawl off the court. I jumped horses until a neurosurgeon told me the next fall might leave me paralyzed. I said to a friend that I thought my first marriage might be in trouble. She looked at me silently for a moment and then said, "Anna, your marriage is over." I stayed in a second marriage for at least a decade too long, to the point the carcass of the dead marriage had turned into bones. I don't know when to quit.

But maybe it's time. It's possible I've run my stretch of this race. It's time to pass the baton. To be honest, I'm tired. I have never seriously thought about quitting before. From the first moment I entered this field, I had a strange sense of certainty that colleagues would come and go, but I was going to be here a while. Thirty-five years later, most of my age cohort have already gone into other lines of work and/or retired, but I have stuck around.

Not all cases go wrong, of course. If they did, I wouldn't be as busy as I am. But when they do go wrong, each one has made a fresh cut that never seems to heal. Enough cuts and you start to bleed just a little too much. Two decades ago, I was unable to prevent two frightened children from being sent back to their sadistic father, and I still see their faces.

It is that sudden, and I know the dam has broken and I am leaving. It will take me several years to extricate myself, but something has shifted, and I'm out of here. I need to spend more time underwater looking at fish.

It would be self-centered to think I was the only problem in that trial. But what I fear most is that it was not technical mistakes on anybody's part that made the difference. The jury just could not comprehend malevolence on that level. He could not be both: the nice, gentle, remorseful man on the stand and the high-risk sex offender I and his therapist painted him out to be. Easier to believe he had reformed. Easier to believe the expert for the defense, who said—as he always does when someone writes a check—that the offender was not high risk to reoffend. After all, crime rates are going down. Not that many sex offenders recidivate. Of course, the "expert" did not remind the jury that this man had already reoffended 19 times after his initial offense.

This sounds as though I think no sex offenders can get better, and that is not what I believe. I could show you 50 to 100 offenders in his program who were at a lower risk to reoffend than he was. But they are making their changes slowly, and they are going to have trouble convincing a jury no matter what they do. They are often nearly illiterate, or toothless, or fall into some ethnic group that white America doesn't trust. They come from poor, dysfunctional backgrounds. They don't speak well. Some are just not that intelligent. Some have brain damage. They don't know the right thing to say or do. This makes it easier to treat them because when they change you can tell. And frankly, their offenses are typically less violent than this man's. But they lack the charm that makes juries forgive all. This man had it.

Chapter 20

Lessons

So, what did I learn by spending over 40 years studying, assessing, and treating sex and other violent offenders? I learned first of all that few people appreciate the variation in sex and violent offender malice and risk. The general public thinks all offenders are the same: "Execution for a first offense," a taxi driver in Dallas told me when he was driving me to a sex abuse conference. But sex offenders range from what I term "lost souls" to "predators" although my experience in the last 15 years has largely been with the latter. They should not all be treated the same as they do not pose the same level of risk, are not driven by the same forces, and do not have the same ability to change their behavior.

Many experts in my field, on the other hand, have become apologists for sex offenders. Most of these experts are kind and decent people who have never assessed or treated a live victim. Victims are an abstraction. The offender they have in front of them is real. He seems pathetic—and many are—raised in horrific environments without the personal resources to be successful in a complex society, although the Jerry Sanduskys and Bill Cosbys of the world do not fall into that category. These experts see society as blaming offenders who were once victims themselves, although most were never victims of sexual abuse. Many offenders falsely claim to have been victims for sympathy (see, for example, Hindman & Peters, 2001). These experts argue that recidivism rates (getting-caught and charged rates) are the same thing as reoffense rates (committing an offense) although the research shows clearly that only 15 percent and 32 percent of offenses are ever reported to authorities and as many as a third of those are never passed from police to prosecutors (see, for example, Daly & Bouhours, 2010). This allows them to argue that instruments that measure recidivism should be used to determine reoffense rates, which serves to understate sex offender risk and let people out of civil commitment programs who should not be released.

Some experts argue that we need to "destigmatize" pedophilia so "these people can get the help they need." My question is if we "destigmatize" pedophilia why would these people think they need help? But in some sense that train has already left the station. *DSM-V*, the diagnostic manual of the American Psychiatric Society, removed pedophilia as a mental disorder in 2012. Only pedophilic disorder is now considered a mental abnormality. For pedophilia to turn into pedophilic disorder, the pedophile has to act on his sexual interest in children (meaning get caught because few who haven't admit to molesting children) or be unhappy being a pedophile. This is one of the only examples in the *DSM-V* where an individual has to commit a crime to have a mental disorder. No one has to act on command hallucinations for them to be a symptom of mental illness, nor does anyone have to object to being schizophrenic to be termed psychotic. What this means is that someone who is quite happy molesting children and does not admit and has not been caught cannot be diagnosed with a mental disorder, even if he is solely attracted to having sex with three-year-olds. It is a political statement, not a scientific one, designed to protect pedophiles from being civilly committed. There has been little, if any, fuss about it.

Recently, I listened to a podcast advising that we be nice to pedophiles and destigmatize a sexual interest in children, which has now been termed a "sexual attraction to minors" to get away from the negative connotations of pedophilia. But pedophilia is the motive for millions of molestations of children. It is a negative. Why should we be trying to whitewash the language? The term "sexually attracted to minors" conflates a sexual interest in post-pubescent 15-year-olds (which is normal although acting on it is a crime) with a sexual

Chapter 20. Lessons

interest in pre-pubescent children, i.e., infants and children up to the age of puberty (which is not normal).

I treat every single offender I have ever interviewed with respect, including serial killers, mass murders, cartel members, psychopaths, and sadists because I believe how we treat people has to do with who we are, not who they are. But that does not mean I believe pedophilia is normal. I don't need to think pedophilia is normal to treat people respectfully. The podcast argued that "only" about 40 percent of molestations are committed by pedophiles which the author said means we should destigmatize it. Forty percent! We should give the green light to the impetus behind a staggering number of child molestations because it is not the only cause of child molestation? Pedophilia is an affliction. Pedophiles may have not chosen it for no one can choose to whom they are sexually attracted, but they are stuck with it and sanitizing it by claiming it is normal only undermines their struggle to control it.

I have also learned that some among us believe everyone can be redeemed and the prodigal son can always return home. They ignore the fact that, as the saying goes, "there are more religious conversions in the back of a patrol car than in church." They believe they don't need to notify the congregation when a church elder who works with children has been found guilty of molesting a child, for example, because all evil is the product of sin, and all one has to do is open one's heart to Christ and all sins are forgiven. Somehow, they think that means the person will not commit more in the future. But having your sins forgiven in the past and being capable of not offending in the future are two different things. It is certainly not just churches who have suffered from the scourge of sexual abuse. Every institution that runs programs for children has had to deal with pedophiles infiltrating their ranks and has been ill-served by naivety and denial among the staff.

But malevolence and malice are real. For those who get a high from hurting others, confession or a claim of religious conversion, even if heartfelt, is not a panacea. Nor do we have the treatment tools to insure that all can be redeemed and that every prodigal son can safely return home. To protect children and ourselves, we must face the fact that we are not human lie detectors and that no, we cannot recognize a sex offender among our families, our friends, our church, and our schools nor tell if one will reoffend. More supervision of the extracurricular activities of our children is needed to combat the sex offenders who hide among coaches, music teachers, tutors, and the like. Our blind belief that nice people are always trustworthy makes our children vulnerable to people with bright smiles and dark thoughts. I have for years thought that if I ever got a tattoo I would put it on my forehead and it would be a quote from Gavin de Becker: "Niceness is a decision, not a character trait" (de Becker, 1997). I have seen the naivete of people who are not sex offenders enable countless sex offenders to obtain access to children, even after being convicted of their crimes.

"I love people who are good and fierce," the four-year-old said from the top of the play structure, brandishing his sword, "but not people who are good, but not fierce." There has to be accountability for sexual offending. Rendering compassion without requiring accountability is a recipe for enabling the continued abuse of children. It's not enough to be good; we have to be fierce in the protection of our children as well.

Finally, from 40 years of work, I have learned to treasure the type of people others take for granted: people who are kind and decent and responsible, who try in ways large and small to make the world a better place, who take care of their children and are kind to their fellow humans. Many times, for example, I have run into people at trainings who have adopted abused children who were damaged beyond total redemption. I feel reverence for the kind of people who will stick with a child who takes a pair of scissors and cuts up all their clothing in their closet. No one notices these people. No one thinks they are heroes. But they are. Kindness is the only god I pledge allegiance to.

Epilogue

> It is a bit embarrassing to have been concerned with the human problem all one's life and find at the end that one has no more to offer by way of advice than "try to be a little kinder."
>
> —Aldous Huxley

Five layers of fleece and wool had seemed sufficient for a day in early October, even at 9500 feet in Colorado, but the wind scouring the plains had cut through all five like a polar bear attacking a salmon. I was freezing. Weather that can kill you feels like a predator stalking prey. I wouldn't have lasted through the night here, even in October. The woman with me had a warm enough coat, but she took off her gloves to feed the frightened and wary mustangs by hand. I decided the gals would have to live with gloves if they wanted the hay I held. My fingers were already stiff inside the gloves. They weren't going to move at all outside them.

The mustangs were recent arrivals, saved from the unpleasant fate that awaited them from the U.S. government. They knew only they had no reason to like people, until the woman had shown up to feed them patiently day by day and haul away the muck and talk quietly to them and slowly make the case for humankind. They were not convinced, but they had become less frightened even though they had only a small corral and not the wide-open plains. There would be time for more room, but for now had she let them out there would have been no way to catch them for vaccines or hoof care or routine vet visits. They needed socializing first. This was The Middle Way, a tiny nonprofit horse sanctuary in

Epilogue

Fairplay, Colorado. Somehow, they had raised the money to buy the mustangs.

I had just met 15 horses, one by one, most of whom except for the three mustangs were broken down, throw-away horses, according to the accounting of the world at large. One had a huge permanent lump in her shoulder area, the results of a broken shoulder. She could not carry the weight of a rider or a foal. What good was she? Another was raised to race but too slow. Besides, her owner had discovered how cruel racing is to horses and had not wanted to be a part of it. Racing is truly not a kind sport, and the horse was traumatized. Another had hoofs that broke down if she was used for riding. She was, apparently, the Bill Walton of the horse world, hoofs not strong enough for her body. There were horses with crooked legs and bad hoofs and bad joints and so many injuries, so very many injuries. One had somehow been impaled on farm equipment and had a deep, permanent indentation in her side. They had injuries that meant they could not be ridden or raced and some could not carry foals or father them. What good were they?

There are more owners than one can count who would have just put them down, but the owners of these horses, many of whom could not afford to keep them, found this place and brought them here. Here they were valued and loved, and their large doe eyes were not frightened or in pain. They were fat and healthy, looked over by a dedicated vet and a trainer/rider both of whom supplemented with their own money what the tiny nonprofit could raise. The vet kept working past the point she wanted to cut back. The trainer had a side customer service job. Neither was paid for taking care of 15 horses. They paid for the horses instead.

Kentucky Thoroughbreds have heated barns and air conditioning in the summer. These horses had a few three-sided shacks, set against the wind. The sanctuary had to raise the money to run electricity out to the mustang corral before winter, the trainer said, or their water would freeze up. (This wasn't winter?)

It was 5 o'clock, and the plains were getting dark. The trainer

Epilogue

moved slowly. Covid had stopped here too, and she was a long hauler with breathing problems, dizziness, brain fog, fatigue, and a host of other symptoms sapping her strength. I once had a single horse to care for in the New Hampshire winter. I was young and strong, and it nearly killed me: getting up every day early and going down to the barn before work to feed and muck manure and break up the frozen water. Every day. There are no days off when you have horses. I had one. They have 15. The trainer's customer service job had placed her on leave. She could not concentrate because of the impact of Covid and kept making mistakes. She said she felt her head was clear but admitted the evidence was everywhere it wasn't. She left tasks and then never remembered to return to them. But here she was, feeding horses, mucking out stalls, talking softly to frightened animals on a bitter cold evening that left me longing for a warm car.

I know grace when I see it. I have a cousin who thinks that Jesus Christ is present in places like this in people like this. I do not share the comfort of belief, but what he calls the presence of Christ I call moments of grace, people of grace. We have different languages, but we see the same thing. These people, who cannot bear to see an animal hurt or discarded or killed for no reason except they are no longer useful to people. These people, who look into the soft, warm eyes of a damaged horse and see a live and loving soul who deserves a chance to live out their days. These people....

At 74, I moved to a cabin at 9300 feet in the Front Range of Colorado, but I continued to work full time for three more years. At 77, I pulled back from my work with sex and violent offenders. Yes, I still give talks and sometimes take cases, but I have spent more time now volunteering at the horse sanctuary and taking pictures for a dog rescue. And there needs to be time for my grown-up children, one of whom lives near me. I like being around kind and purposeful people. I have served my time with the malevolent, the confused, and the callous. I ride my Lusitano dressage horse, and I take my German Shepherd to a creek every day in the summer and throw 50 sticks in the water one by one. To retrieve them, she launches herself into the water with giant bellyflops.

The only two things that get better as we get older are an appreciation of beauty and the ability to be kind. Strangely, noticing beauty will make you kinder. If you are getting older and you aren't getting kinder, something is wrong with the way you are living your life. But if you are reading this, there is still time.

I am 78 now. A grandchild and a white horse have drawn me from my beloved Colorado mountains to Tennessee. Each morning, I get up before the sun rises, grab a cup of coffee, prop myself up in bed, and wait for the coming of the light, until the pattern of the windowpanes lies in glory across my sheets. The coming of the light is worth waiting for, each and every day.

Then I rise and go to see the white horse. I go down in the meadow to fetch him, armed with apples or carrots or his favorite, watermelon, and together Al and I walk up through the long, green pasture. OK, I walk and Al glides, but we get there. I whisper on the way he is the most handsome horse who ever lived, but Al is modest and doesn't comment. I brush his silky fur and clean his small, neat hoofs, and saddle him. We go into the covered arena with the exacting instructor who yells at both of us, criticism and praise, but who keeps him supple and me learning. We passage, and we piaffe, and we canter in the rocking horse way that dressage horses do.

In the arena I am no longer old and creaky; I have grown four strong legs and powerful haunches that catapult me across the arena. I dance with the most sensitive of partners: twist one way and he turns that way, twist the other way and again he turns, lay a leg on his side and off he goes sideways, both front and back legs crossing over. What do hands have to do with it? I would not insult Al by waterskiing on his face. For a long time, I rode him without a bit. My way was long and crooked to Al's back, but now his back is home.

Find your white horse, even if he isn't a white horse. Find the coming of the light, even if it is not at dawn. Light and white horses will make you kind, and kindness brings peace.

Chapter Notes

Introduction

1. Reprinted by the permission of The Charlotte Sheedy Literary Agency as agent for the author. Copyright © 1990, 2006, 2008, 2017 by Mary Oliver with permission of Bill Reichblum.

2. Yes, there are female offenders, but the majority are male, and certainly the overwhelming number of sex offenders that I have interviewed in prison or civil commitment programs are male. Therefore, for convenience I will use male pronouns to describe offenders. I have had little experience with female sex offenders.

Chapter 1

1. Generally, evidence is thrown out when a judge rules it is more prejudicial than probative. This means that it is thought to pose an intolerable risk to the fairness of the proceedings or reliability of the outcome. Juries are often not allowed to hear that a defendant has committed this type of crime before because then, for an example, anyone with a history of any particular type of crime, e.g., child molestation, would be easy to convict if accused of that type of crime again. There are exceptions to this law and times that "prior bad acts" are admitted as evidence.

2. I tried hard to find a more dignified term, but sometimes a pissing match is a pissing match.

Chapter 2

1. He divorced his wife and married her. Against all odds, they stayed together for the rest of their lives.

2. Pete Maravich became a professional basketball player who was inducted into the Basketball Hall of Fame after his career ended. His jersey was retired by three teams that he played for.

Chapter 3

1. He was tried as an adult, even though the offense was committed when he was 17. Thus, the trial was public, my testimony was public, and even my report was released to the press. Therefore, I am able to talk about any aspects already in the public domain.

Chapter 4

1. My mother's real name was Rosalie, but for some reason my father didn't like that name and always called her Kate.

2. When the new county hospital was built, the departments were each named for one of the early doctors who worked there in the late '40s on up and who made house calls to the far reaches of the county for decades before reinforcements arrived.

Chapter 6

1. Of course, these aren't all of the defenses. One psychopath raped his

Chapter Notes

therapist after convincing her he had multiple personalities, then claimed one of his alters raped her. He was charming enough that she testified for him. The problem was, he had no history of dissociative identity disorder (multiple personalities) and a long history of psychopathy. Neither the prosecutor nor, more importantly, the jury was impressed with his "alters."

Chapter 10

1. True story of a religious sect in Wisconsin. Unfortunately, they're all true stories.

Chapter 12

1. Yes, indeed, if you are a sailor, you are wondering what the hell we were doing in Woods Hole in the middle of the night with no motor, no radio, and no radar. Four words: young, stupid, and broke.

Chapter 14

1. All names have been changed in this and every episode to protect the guilty.

2. Not saying I understand that one.
3. True example of an elementary school child already wildly off the normal track. He later went on to shoot his father in the head in the middle of the night at age 12.
4. Of course, this example depends on a community's collective experience with the police as either basically fair, impartial law enforcers or arbitrary, hostile oppressors.
5. Ironically, some people with PTSD also misread the intentions of others but it is through fear and without the anger and propensity for violence of offenders.

Chapter 19

1. Example from a therapist report of an actual case of physical abuse of an infant in which the man later killed the child. The infant had bites all over his body when the psychologist saw him.
2. If you doubt this, look up octopus camouflage on YouTube. With a little hunting you can find an astounding video of an octopus who looks exactly like seaweed until the photographer gets close and scares the octopus into fleeing.

Bibliography

Angelou, M. (1991). *All God's Children Need Traveling Shoes.* Vintage Books.
Berg, R. (2011). Parental alienation analysis, domestic violence, and gender bias in Minnesota courts. *Law and Inequity, 29*(5), 5–31.
Brown, T., Frederico, M., Hewitt, L., & Sheehan, R. (1997). Problems and solutions in the management of child abuse allegations in custody and access disputes in the family court. *Family and Conciliation Courts Review36, 36*(4), 431–443.
Bruch, C. (2001). Parental alienation and parental alienation syndrome: Getting it wrong in child custody cases. *Family Law Quarterly, 35*(3), 527–552.
Cialdini, R.B. (2001). *Influence: Science and Practice.* Allyn & Bacon.
Clemente, M., & Padilla-Racero, D. (2016). When courts accept what science rejects: Custody issues concerning the alleged "parental alienation syndrome." *Journal of Child Custody, 13*(2–3), 126–133.
Dallam, S.J., & Silberg, J.L. (2016). Recommended treatments for "parental alienation syndrome" (PAS) may cause children foreseeable and lasting psychological harm. *Journal of Child Custody, 13*(2–3), 134–143.
Dalton, C., Drozd, L., & Wong, F. (2006). *Navigating Custody and Visitation Evaluations in Cases of Domestic Violence: A Judge's Guide.* National Council of Juvenile and Family Court Judges.
Daly, M., & Bouhours, B. (2010). Rape and attrition in the legal process: A comparative analysis of five countries. *Crime and Justice, 39*, 565–650.
de Becker, G. (1997). *The Gift of Fear.* Little, Brown.
De Botton, A. (2006). *The Architecture of Happiness.* Vintage House.
Dillard, A. (1974). *Pilgrim at Tinker Creek.* Bantam Books.
Doyle, A.C. (1892). The Adventure of the Cooper Beeches. In *The Adventures of Sherlock Holmes.* George Newnes.
Einstein, A. (1934). *Einstein Essays in Science.* Dover Publications.
Erickson, M.F. (2017). *In the Room with Milton Erickson.* Jane Parsons-Fein Training Institute.
Faller, K.C. (1998). The parental alienation syndrome: What is it and what data support it. *Child Maltreatment, 3*(2), 100–115.
Gardner, R.A. (1987). *The Parental Alienation Syndrome and the Differentiation Between Fabricated and Genuine Child Sex Abuse.* Creative Therapeutics.
Gardner, R.A. (1992). *True and False Allegations of Child Sexual Abuse.* Creative Therapeutics.
Gardner, R.A. (2000). Family therapy of the moderate type of parental alienation syndrome. *The American Journal of Family Therapy, 27*, 195–212.
Gardner, R.A. (2002). The role of the judiciary in the entrenchment of the parental alienation syndrome (PAS). https://childrightsngo.com/newdownload/downloadsection8/PAS%20and%20Role%20of%20Judiciary.pdf.

Bibliography

Hindman, J., & Peters, J. (2001). Polygraph testing leads to better understanding adult and juvenile sex offenders. *Federal Probation, 65*(3), 8–15.

Hoult, J. (2006). The evidentiary admissibility of parental alienation syndrome: Science, law, and policy. *Children's Legal Rights Journal, 26*(1), 1–61.

Huff, S.C. (2015). *Expanding the relationship between parental alienating behaviors and children's contact refusal following divorce: Testing additional factors and long-term outcomes.* University of Connecticut.

Keillor, G. (1982). *We Are Still Married.* Viking Penguin.

King, S. (1982). *Rita Hayworth and the Shawshank Redemption.* Simon & Schuster.

Leopold, A. (1949). *A Sand Country Almanac and Sketches Here and There.* Oxford University Press.

London, Kamala, Burck, Maggie, Ceci, Stephen, and Shuman, Daniel W. (2005) Disclosures of child sexual abuse: What does the research tell us about the ways that children tell. *Psychology, Public Practice, and the Law,* 11(1), pp. 194-226

Maruna, S. (2001). *Making Good: How Ex-Convicts Reform and Rebuild Their Lives.* American Psychological Association.

Meier, J. (2009). A historical perspective on parental alienation syndrome and parental alienation. *Journal of Child Custody, 6i*232–257.

Meier, J.S., & Dickson, S. (2017). Mapping gender: Shedding empirical light on family courts' treatment of cases involving abuse and alienation. *Law & Inequality: A Journal of Theory and Practice, 35*(2), 311–334.

Michaud, S.G., & Aynesworth, H. (1989). *Ted Bundy: Conversations with a Killer.* Penguin.

Neilson, L.C. (2018). *Parental alienation empirical analysis: Child best interest or parental rights?* https://www.fredacentre.com/wp-content/uploads/Parental-Alienation-Linda-Neilson.pdf.

O'Donohue, W., Benuto, L., & Bennett, N. (2016). Examining the validity of parental alienation syndrome. *Journal of Child Custody, 13*(2–3), 113–125.

Rüdiger, T.-G. (2015). *The real world on online gaming and sexual predators.* http://www.beakidshero.com/posts/the-real-world-of-sexual-predators-and-online-gaming.

Rush, F. (1980). *The Best Kept Secret: Sexual Abuse of Children.* McGraw-Hill.

Salter, A.C. (1988). *Treating Child Sex Offenders and Victims: A Practical Guide.* Sage.

Schuman, R. (2000). Allegations of sexual abuse. In P. Stah (Ed.), *Complex Issues in Child Custody Evaluations.* Sage.

Shire, W. (2015). *Facing History & Ourselves, "'Home' by Warsan Shire."* https://www.facinghistory.org/resource-library/home-warsan-shire.

Slabach, M.A. (2014). Today's estranged child; yesterday's alienating parent? *ACFS Family Law Specialist, 3,* 8–11.

Stevens, W. (1990). Man Carrying Thing. In *The Collected Poems of Wallace Stevens.* Alfred A. Knopf.

Thoennes, N., & Tjaden, P.G. (1990). The extent, nature, and validity of sexual abuse allegations in custody/visitation disputes. *Child Abuse and Neglect: The International Journal, 14,* 151–163.

Thomas, R.M., & Richardson, J.T. (2015). 30 years on and still junk science. *The Judges' Journal, 54*(3), 22–24.

Wallerstein, J., & Kelly, J. (1980). *Surviving the Breakup: How Children and Parents Cope with Divorce.* Basic Books.

Wallerstein, J., Lewis, J., & Blakeslee, S. (2001). *The Unexpected Legacy of Divorce: A 25 Year Landmark Study.* Basic Books.

www.ingramcontent.com/pod-product-compliance
Ingram Content Group UK Ltd.
Pitfield, Milton Keynes, MK11 3LW, UK
UKHW042011140426
5217IPUK00015B/1111